Pharmaceutical Calculations Workbook

Pharmaceutical Calculations Workbook

Judith A Rees

BPharm, MSc, PhD, MRPharmS
Senior Lecturer
School of Pharmacy and Pharmaceutical Sciences
University of Manchester, UK

Ian Smith

BSc, MRPharmS
Boots Teacher Practitioner
School of Pharmacy and Pharmaceutical Sciences
University of Manchester, UK

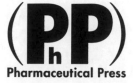

Pharmaceutical Press

Published by the Pharmaceutical Press

66-68 East Smithfield, London E1W 1AW, UK

© Pharmaceutical Press 2006

(P.P) is a trade mark of Pharmaceutical Press

Pharmaceutical Press is the publishing division of the Royal
Pharmaceutical Society of Great Britain

First published 2006
Reprinted 2008, 2009, 2010, 2011, 2013, 2014, 2015, 2016, 2017, 2020, 2021

Typeset by TypeStudy, Scarborough, North Yorkshire
Printed in Great Britain by TJ Books Ltd, Padstow, Cornwall

ISBN 978 0 85369 602 5

A catalogue record for this book is available from the British Library.

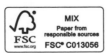

Contents

Preface

There is a saying that 'practice makes perfect'. Well, we are not saying that practising pharmaceutical calculations will make you perfect, but practising will:

- give you experience in dealing with the myriad of types of pharmaceutical calculations
- enable you to sort out easily the way to tackle the question
- give you confidence with calculations
- make you quicker at solving the problems
- make you more able to arrive at the correct answer every time.

This workbook, as a companion volume to *Introduction to Pharmaceutical Calculations*, was written in response to the frequent demands from pharmacy students, preregistration trainees and their trainers for more examples to practise. We know from the many comments we have received that *Introduction to Pharmaceutical Calculations* showed how to do the various pharmaceutical calculations and gave some examples for practice, but readers just wanted more and more examples to practise. And so the idea of a workbook was born.

The workbook gives many more examples for the reader to practice than could possibly be incorporated into *Introduction to Pharmaceutical Calculations*. The two books should be used together since the workbook relies on *Introduction to Pharmaceutical Calculations* to explain the methods used to tackle the calculations. For the convenience of the reader, the topics covered in the chapters in the workbook correspond to the chapters in *Introduction to Pharmaceutical Calculations*, so readers having difficulty with a particular type of calculation or requiring more examples for practice can turn to the corresponding chapter in the companion volume.

The layout of each chapter is similar. Basic concepts are presented in tables with spaces to be completed by the reader. These tables set out the information in a clear way and require the reader to calculate further information. Practice with these tables should indicate to the reader that there is a relationship between pieces of information. Thus, in calculations the starting point (e.g. concentration of solution) may be given and the reader asked to calculate the final answer (e.g. concentration of the final solution) or the final answer (e.g. required dose) given and the amount of starting point (e.g. amount of available formulation) calculated. Realisation that questions can be asked that require the reader to sort out and reorder information in order to calculate the correct answer will help with the more complex questions elsewhere in each chapter. These more complex questions may include specific drugs, formulations and doses and are usually, although not always, patient related. These questions require the reader to sort out the information given in order to calculate the correct answer. In questions requiring the knowledge of specific dosage regimens, composition of formulations, rates of delivery, etc., the information is given, rather than expecting the reader to look up this information.

Answers to all the tables and questions are provided at the end of each chapter.

Whilst some readers may start at the beginning and go through to the end, it is expected that most readers will not. It is recommended that readers start with the tables, but where a reader is confident in that type of calculation (and we are all different in the types of calculations that appear easy to us individually) then they should complete as much of the tables as suits their needs and go onto the next question, and so on.

Next to the vexed question of whether the reader requires or should use a calculator. Obviously it is the reader's choice, but the Royal Pharmaceutical Society does not allow the use of calculators in their Registration Examination and so most preregistration trainees would be wise to attempt the calculations without a calculator. All the questions in the workbook can be attempted without the use of a calculator, although some questions, especially those involving molecular weights, may pose some challenges. With these questions it is suggested that the reader approximates the values, e.g. a molecular weight of 289 can be approximated to 300 and the answer worked out without a calculator to obtain an approximate answer. This approximate answer will be in the right order of magnitude and very similar to the correct answer. If the answer obtained is about the same as the answer at the end of the chapter, then the reader can be assured that they have used the correct method to work out the answer. The true value of the answer can always be checked using a calculator.

Finally, we hope that this workbook will satisfy all the requests we have received for 'more and more examples for practice' and that, indeed, practice will go some way to make you perfect!

Judith A Rees and Ian Smith
Manchester, July 2005

About the authors

Judith A Rees is a senior lecturer in the School of Pharmacy at the University of Manchester, where she lectures and researches in the area of pharmacy practice. Additionally, she is, and has been in the recent past, external examiner in pharmacy practice to several UK schools of pharmacy. She is a registered pharmacist.

Ian Smith is a Boots Teacher Practitioner, which combines being a pharmacist with Boots The Chemists and teaching pharmacy practice in the School of Pharmacy and Pharmaceutical Sciences at the University of Manchester.

How to use this workbook

This workbook was designed as a companion volume to *Introduction to Pharmaceutical Calculations*. The aim of the workbook was to provide many more examples than could be offered in *Introduction to Pharmaceutical Calculations* and so give readers the opportunity to obtain more practice with pharmaceutical calculations.

It was anticipated that readers would use both volumes together and for this reason the order in which topics and chapters are presented is the same for both books. Thus, if a reader has any difficulty performing one or more of the calculations in the workbook, then it is suggested that the reader refers to the appropriate chapter or chapters in *Introduction to Pharmaceutical Calculations* to sort out the basic techniques and approaches to solving the calculation. Because the chapters and hence topic areas follow the same order in both books, it is easy if the reader feels competent in calculations for a particular topic area for these topics to be deliberately missed out and the next chapter or topic area tackled.

Each chapter consists of tables for completion and individual, often drug- or patient-specific, questions. The tables are designed for the reader to practise basic calculation skills. It is not necessary for the reader to complete all of a table if they feel confident in their abilities at that type of calculation. Some of the tables are useful for demonstrating how component parts of a more complex problem can be separated out. Completing these tables may prepare the reader for tackling more complex and specific calculations.

The workbook is laid out such that the questions are placed on the left-hand page and the opposite right-hand page is left free for 'working out'. After working through a calculation on the right-hand page the reader should inset the answer in the space provided on the left-hand page. Calculations involving tables will have spaces left in the table for the reader to fill in with their answer, whereas individual questions have a defined space for the answer.

After completing a table or specific questions, the reader may check their answer with the correct answer. All the answers to calculations in a chapter are found at the end of the chapter.

1

Calculations involving rational numbers

LEARNING OBJECTIVES

Questions in this chapter cover the following:

- deciding if sets of numbers are proportional or non-proportional
- finding the missing numerator or denominator for a fraction
- expressing fractions in their lowest terms
- multiplication of fractions
- expressing numbers as decimals, fractions or percentages
- finding the missing value in proportional sets and setting up proportional sets

Q1 State whether the following sets of numbers are proportional or non-proportional. If the set is proportional, state the ratio for the set.

A	2	4	6	8	
	36	72	108	144	-----------------------------

B	12	14	16	
	30	32	36	-----------------------------

C	25	49	81	
	5	7	9	-----------------------------

D	24	30	36	
	6	7.5	9	-----------------------------

E	3	27	32	
	1.5	13.5	18	-----------------------------

F	25	26	27	
	28	29	30	-----------------------------

NOTES

G   2.4   5.9

     48   118   ------------------------------

H   1.25   2.5   3.75

     4.5   5.0   5.5   ------------------------------

I   101   106

     11   16   ------------------------------

J   40   50   60

     70   80   90   ------------------------------

K   40   50   60

     48   60   72   ------------------------------

L   102   122

     40.8   48.8   ------------------------------

M   105   112

     1155   1232   ------------------------------

N   0.87   0.918

     4.35   4.59   ------------------------------

O   136   106

     13.6   11.6   ------------------------------

Q2   Calculate the numerator of the fraction that is equal to the stated fraction with the denominator shown.

	Fraction	Numerator	Denominator
A	1/8	---------------	40
B	1/7	---------------	56
C	2/3	---------------	21
D	15/300	---------------	20

NOTES

E	15/21	---------------	7
F	14/114	---------------	342
G	18/3	---------------	39
H	121/11	---------------	1
I	2/82	---------------	205
J	4/16	---------------	20

Q3 Calculate the denominator of the fraction that is equal to the stated fraction with the numerator shown.

	Fraction	Numerator	Denominator
A	12/36	144	---------------
B	84/6	42	---------------
C	1/16	8	---------------
D	6/90	9	---------------
E	13/15	52	---------------
F	2/5	22	---------------
G	4/9	36	---------------
H	136/200	17	---------------
I	56/72	7	---------------
J	9/81	1	---------------

Q4 Express the following fractions in their lowest terms:

A   3/27   ---------------

B   124/336   ---------------

NOTES

C   27/36   ----------------

D   45/60   ----------------

E   36/2880   ----------------

F   42/49   ----------------

G   121/99   ----------------

H   13/117   ----------------

I   68/336   ----------------

J   1610/3266   ----------------

Q5   Express the answers to the following multiplications as fractions in their lowest terms:

A $5/9 \times 21 =$ ----------------

B $1/3 \times 5 =$ ----------------

C $2/21 \times 6 =$ ----------------

D $3/8 \times 12 =$ ----------------

E $2/45 \times 9 =$ ----------------

F $32/90 \times 3 =$ ----------------

G $64/1245 \times 15 =$ ----------------

H $12/81 \times 18 =$ ----------------

I $42/49 \times 1.5 =$ ----------------

J $32/136 \times 3.5 =$ ----------------

NOTES

Q6   Convert the following fractions to decimals (state two places) and percentages:

	Fraction	Decimal	Percentage
A	1/4	---------------	---------------
B	1/7	---------------	---------------
C	7/8	---------------	---------------
D	19/25	---------------	---------------
E	2/9	---------------	---------------
F	56/12	---------------	---------------
G	60/50	---------------	---------------
H	1/16	---------------	---------------
I	9/81	---------------	---------------
J	124/900	---------------	---------------
K	15/32	---------------	---------------
L	3/14	---------------	---------------
M	14/15	---------------	---------------
N	3/13	---------------	---------------
O	1/25	---------------	---------------
P	8/9	---------------	---------------
Q	7/10	---------------	---------------
R	7/16	---------------	---------------
S	7/32	---------------	---------------

NOTES

Q7   Convert the following decimals to percentages and fractions (expressed in the lowest terms):

	Decimal	Percentage	Fraction
A	0.56	----------------	----------------
B	0.135	----------------	----------------
C	0.77	----------------	----------------
D	0.015	----------------	----------------
E	0.103 4	----------------	----------------
F	0.937 5	----------------	----------------
G	2.35	----------------	----------------
H	37.5	----------------	----------------
I	0.375	----------------	----------------
J	0.45	----------------	----------------
K	0.32	----------------	----------------
L	0.085	----------------	----------------
M	0.312 5	----------------	----------------
N	0.056	----------------	----------------
O	0.42	----------------	----------------
P	5.6	----------------	----------------
Q	0.89	----------------	----------------
R	0.562 5	----------------	----------------
S	0.755	----------------	----------------

NOTES

Q8   Express the following percentages as decimals and fractions (expressed in lowest terms):

	Percentage	Decimal	Fraction
A	40%	---------------	---------------
B	60%	---------------	---------------
C	52%	---------------	---------------
D	27%	---------------	---------------
E	5.5%	---------------	---------------
F	16.25%	---------------	---------------
G	101.2%	---------------	---------------
H	0.05%	---------------	---------------
I	10.025%	---------------	---------------
J	25.34%	---------------	---------------
K	45.25%	---------------	---------------
L	76.5%	---------------	---------------
M	0.75%	---------------	---------------
N	45.32%	---------------	---------------
O	56.8%	---------------	---------------
P	16.6%	---------------	---------------
Q	109.7%	---------------	---------------
R	67.2%	---------------	---------------
S	44.28%	---------------	---------------

NOTES

Q9   Find the missing values from the following proportional sets:

A   21   -----
     42   84

B   8   20
     2   -----

C   2   -----   16
     24   36   -----

D   16   17
     40   -----

E   190   210
     ----- 16.8

F   155   25
     31   -----

G   ----- 28
     45   70

H   216   296
     ----- 370

I   15   -----
     22.5 576

J   3   168
     12.3 -----

K   14   -----
     16   45

L   35   -----   1610
     ----- 3053   3220

NOTES

M   0.4   0.8

-----   0.4

N   -----   7.2   8.4

0.4   0.6   -----

O   3.5   192.5

-----   231

P   516   -----   1290

-----   154.8   258

Q   0.2   -----

0.028   0.016 8

R   -----   0.021

0.7   0.14

S   1/2   1/8

4   -----

T   3/4   -----

1/8   1/4

Q10 Set up the following proportional sets.

A   A lorry travels at 45 mph. Set up the proportional sets for the distance travelled every half hour from 0 to 3 hours.

B   Digoxin tablets contain 0.0625 mg per tablet. Set up the proportional sets for the amount of digoxin contained in 0 to 5 tablets.

NOTES

C   A patient takes one tablet twice a day. Set up the proportional set for the number of tablets you need to dispense for each week's supply for up to 4 weeks.

D   Each Fersaday tablet contains 322 mg of ferrous fumarate. How much ferrous fumarate is contained in 10 tablets?

E   25 g of ointment contains 7 g of zinc oxide. How much zinc oxide will be contained in 100 g of ointment?

F   A patient takes 15 mL of medicine per day. How much would you need to dispense for a month's supply?

G   1 L of medicine contains 125 mL of alcohol. How much alcohol is contained in 100 mL of medicine?

H   Amoxicillin is dispensed as 125 mg/5 mL syrup. How much amoxicillin is there in 100 mL of syrup?

I   Tobramycin should be given at a dose of 2 mg/kg every 12 hours in a neonate. What would be the dose every 12 hours for a neonate weighing 3.0 kg?

J   30 g of cream contains 7.5 g of drug x. What is the amount of cream that contains 97.5 g of drug x?

NOTES

ANSWERS

A1   **A**   Proportional in the ratio 1:18

        B   Not proportional

        C   Not proportional

        D   Proportional in the ratio 4:1

        E   Not proportional

        F   Not proportional

        G   Proportional in the ratio 1:20

        H   Not proportional

        I   Not proportional

        J   Not proportional

        K   Proportional in the ratio 1:1.2

        L   Proportional in the ratio 2.5:1

        M   Proportional in the ratio 1:11

        N   Proportional in the ratio 1:5

        O   Not proportional

A2   **A**   5

        B   8

        C   14

        D   1

        E   5

        F   42

        G   234

        H   11

        I   5

        J   5

A3   **A**   432

        B   3

        C   128

D   135

E   60

F   55

G   81

H   25

I   9

J   9

A4   **A**   1/9

B   31/84

C   3/4

D   3/4

E   1/80

F   6/7

G   11/9

H   1/9

I   17/84

J   805/1633

A5   **A**   105/9 = 35/3

B   5/3

C   12/21 = 4/7

D   36/8 = 9/2

E   18/45 = 2/5

F   96/90 = 16/15

G   960/1245 = 64/83

H   216/81 = 8/3

I   63/49 = 9/7

J   112/136 = 14/17

A6

	Decimal	Percentage
A	0.25	25%
B	0.14	14.29%
C	0.88	87.5%
D	0.76	76%
E	0.22	22.22%
F	4.67	466.67%
G	1.2	120%
H	0.06	6.25%
I	0.11	11.11%
J	0.14	13.78%
K	0.47	46.88%
L	0.21	21.43%
M	0.93	93.33%
N	0.23	23.08%
O	0.04	4%
P	0.89	88.89%
Q	0.70	70%
R	0.44	43.75%
S	0.22	21.88%

A7

	Percentage	Fraction
A	56%	56/100 = 14/25
B	13.5%	135/1000 = 27/200
C	77%	77/100
D	1.5%	15/1000 = 3/200
E	10.34%	1034/10 000 = 517/5000
F	93.75%	9375/10 000 = 15/16
G	235%	235/100 = 47/20

H	3750%	375/10 = 75/2
I	37.5%	375/1000 = 3/8
J	45%	45/100 = 9/20
K	32%	32/100 = 8/25
L	8.5%	85/1000 = 17/200
M	31.25%	3125/10 000 = 5/16
N	5.6%	56/1000 = 7/125
O	42%	42/100 = 21/50
P	560%	56/10 = 28/5
Q	89%	89/100
R	56.25%	5625/1000 = 3/4
S	75.5%	755/1000 = 151/200

A8

	Decimal	*Fraction*
A	0.4	40/100 = 2/5
B	0.6	60/100 = 3/5
C	0.52	52/100 = 13/25
D	0.27	27/100
E	0.055	55/1000 = 11/200
F	0.162 5	1625/10 000 = 13/80
G	1.012	1012/1000 = 253/250
H	0.000 5	5/10 000 = 1/2000
I	0.100 25	10 025/100 000 = 401/4000
J	0.253 4	2534/10 000 = 1267/5000
K	0.452 5	4525/10 000 = 181/400
L	0.765	765/1000 = 153/200
M	0.007 5	75/10 000 = 3/400
N	0.453 2	4532/10 000 = 1133/2500
O	0.568	568/1000 = 71/125
P	0.166	166/1000 = 83/500

Q	1.097	1097/1000
R	0.672	672/1000 = 84/125
S	0.442 8	4428/10 000 = 1107/2500

A9

A	42	
B	5	
C	3, 192	
D	42.5	
E	15.2	
F	5	
G	18	
H	270	
I	384	
J	688.8	
K	39.375	
L	70, 1526.5	
M	0.2	
N	4.8, 0.7	
O	4.2	
P	103.2, 774	
Q	0.12	
R	0.105	
S	1	
T	3/2 = 1.5	

A10   **A**

Distance travelled (miles)	0	22.5	45	67.5	90	112.5	135
Time (hours)	0	0.5	1	1.5	2	2.5	3

B

Number of tablets	0	1	2	3	4	5
Amount of digoxin (mg)	0	0.0625	0.125	0.1875	0.25	0.3125

C

Number of weeks	1	2	3	4
Number of tablets	14	28	42	56

D

Let the amount of ferrous fumarate in 10 tablets = a

Number of Fersaday tablets	1	10
Amount of ferrous furmarate (mg)	322	a

E

Let the amount of zinc oxide in 100 g = x

Amount of zinc oxide (g)	7	x
Amount of ointment (g)	25	100

F

Let the amount dispensed in a month = x

Amount of medicine (mL)	15	x
Number of days	1	28

G

Let the amount of alcohol in 100 mL of medicine = x

Amount of alcohol (mL)	125	x
Amount of medicine (mL)	1000	100

H

Let the amount of amoxicillin in 100 mL = y

Amount of amoxicillin (mg)	125	y
Amount of syrup (mL)	5	100

I

Let the dose of tobramycin every 12 hours for the neonate = z

Dose of tobramycin every 12 hours (mg)	2	z
Weight (kg)	1	3.0

J

Let the amount of cream containing 97.5 g = x

Amount of cream (g)	30	x
Amount of drug x (g)	7.5	97.5

2

Calculations involving systems of units

LEARNING OBJECTIVES

Questions in this chapter cover the following:
- converting and manipulating different expressions within the metric system
- converting between imperial and metric units

Changing metric units

Q1   Complete the following:

A   223 mg   = _____ g   = _____ kg   = _____ micrograms

B   32 mg   = _____ g   = _____ kg   = _____ micrograms

C   45.6 mg   = _____ g   = _____ kg   = _____ micrograms

D   0.003 52 mg   = _____ g   = _____ micrograms = _____ nanograms

E   0.000 59 mg   = _____ micrograms = _____ nanograms   = _____ picograms

F   1.2 mg   = _____ micrograms = _____ nanograms   = _____ g

G   250 micrograms   = _____ mg   = _____ nanograms   = _____ g

H   6000 micrograms = _____ mg   = _____ nanograms   = _____ g

I   1.3 kg   = _____ g   = _____ mg   = _____ micrograms

J   0.6 kg   = _____ g   = _____ mg   = _____ micrograms

K   0.000 546 kg   = _____ g   = _____ mg   = _____ micrograms

L   57 g   = _____ kg   = _____ mg

NOTES

M   8.67 g   = _____ kg   = _____ mg

N   250 nanograms   = _____ mg   = _____ micrograms

O   0.152 nanograms = _____ mg   = _____ micrograms = _____ picograms

Q2   Complete the following:

A   10 mL   = _____ L   = _____ microlitres

B   420 mL   = _____ L   = _____ microlitres

C   2.13 L   = _____ mL

D   0.000 95 L   = _____ mL = _____ microlitres

E   23 000 microlitres = _____ mL = _____ L

Q3   Complete the following:

A   1700 mm   = _____ cm = _____ m   = _____ micrometres

B   0.78 mm   = _____ cm = _____ m   = _____ micrometres

C   1.25 mm   = _____ cm = _____ m   = _____ micrometres

D   0.25 cm   = _____ mm = _____ m

E   15.6 cm   = _____ mm = _____ m

F   0.064 cm   = _____ mm = _____ m

G   1.2 m   = _____ cm = _____ m

H   13 m   = _____ cm = _____ mm

I   0.008 9 m   = _____ cm = _____ mm = _____ micrometres

J   9056 micrometres = _____ m   = _____ cm = _____ mm

NOTES

Q4   Add the following:

    A   3.09 g + 15 000 mg + 16 500 000 micrograms   = _____ g

    B   1.095 kg + 446.07 g + 10 780 mg   = _____ g

    C   1 mg + 56 000 micrograms + 150 000 nanograms = _____ micrograms

    D   0.125 mg + 275 micrograms + 9.578 65 g   = _____ mg

    E   112 mL + 0.098 L   = _____ mL

    F   1.5 L + 9548 mL   = _____ L

    G   18.876 mm + 0.925 cm + 5687 micrometres   = _____ mm

    H   324 cm + 6.571 m + 19 000 mm   = _____ cm

    I   700 000 mm + 54 679.9 cm + 0.578 45 m   = _____ mm

    J   0.89 m + 1700 cm + 86 000 mm   = _____ m

Q5   A pharmacist dispenses 150 mg and 620 mg of a drug from a container containing 5 g. How many grams are left in the container?

    _____ g

Q6   A pharmacists measures out three amounts of 200 mL and two amounts of 150 mL from a stock bottle of 2 L. How many millilitres are left in the stock bottle?

    _____ mL

Q7   A patient receives 500 nanograms of alfacalcidol each day for 30 days. How much alfacalcidol does the patient receive in the 30 days, expressed as milligrams?

    _____ mg

Q8   What amount in microlitres of peppermint oil would be contained in each capsule, if 50 mL of peppermint oil is used to manufacture 50 000 capsules?

    _____ microlitres

NOTES

Q9   If 125 000 capsules can be made from 0.425 kg of ibuprofen, how many capsules can be made from 850 g?

Q10   A beclometasone inhaler contains 200 doses per unit and each metered dose contains 50 micrograms of beclometasone dipropionate. How many milligrams of beclometasone dipropionate are there in each 200 dose unit?

-------------- mg

Q11   Kliovance tablets contain estradiol 1 mg and norethisterone acetate 500 micrograms. How many grams of estradiol and norethisterone acetate are there in a packet of 28 tablets?

-------------- g estradiol

-------------- g norethisterone acetate

Q12   A tablet is 4.2 mm thick. What is the height in centimetres of a stack of 25 tablets?

-------------- cm

Q13   How many litres of solution are required to fill 300 bottles each containing 250 mL?

-------------- L

Q14   Folic acid 400-microgram tablets come in containers of 90 tablets. How many milligrams of folic acid are there in a container?

-------------- mg

Q15   A patch contains 7.5 mg of drug x. How much of drug x is contained in 30 patches, expressed as grams?

-------------- g

NOTES

Changing units between different systems of measurement

The answers are based on the conversion factors in Appendix 2, *Introduction to Pharmaceutical Calculations*, 2nd edn.

Q16   Convert the following:

A   2 L   = _____ pints   or _____ pints _____ fluid ounces

B   0.76 L = _____ pints   or _____ pints _____ fluid ounces

C   70 L   = _____ gallons or _____ gallons _____ pints _____ fluid ounces

D   300 mL = _____ fluid ounces

E   721 mL = _____ pints _____ fluid ounces

Q17   Convert the following:

A   10 pints   = _____ L

B   6 gallons   = _____ L

C   10 fluid ounces   = _____ mL

D   1 gallon 3 pints   = _____ L

E   2 gallons 5 pints 6 fluid ounces = _____ L

Q18   Convert the following:

A   2.6 kg   = _____ pounds

B   140 kg   = _____ pounds or _____ stone _____ pounds

C   4000 g   = _____ pounds or _____ pounds _____ ounces

D   769 000 mg = _____ ounces

E   76.89 g   = _____ ounces

NOTES

Q19   Convert the following:

   A   621 ounces   = _____ g

   B   452 pounds   = _____ kg

   C   8 stone 6 pounds   = _____ kg

   D   2 pounds 6 ounces   = _____ kg

   E   12 stone 11 pounds 7 ounces = _____ g = _____ kg

Q20   Convert the following:

   A   6 feet   = _____ m

   B   10 inches   = _____ cm

   C   15 yards   = _____ m

   D   21 miles   = _____ km

   E   5 feet 4 inches = _____ m

Q21   Convert the following:

   A   1.22 m   = _____ feet   or _____ feet _____ inches

   B   36 cm   = _____ inches

   C   350 m   = _____ yards or _____ yards _____ feet _____ inches

   D   1.74 m   = _____ feet   or _____ feet _____ inches

   E   1795 mm = _____ inches

Q22   Convert the following:

   A   16 degrees Celsius   = _____ degrees Fahrenheit

   B   101 degrees Celsius   = _____ degrees Fahrenheit

   C   37.5 degrees Celsius   = _____ degrees Fahrenheit

NOTES

D   −30 degrees Celsius   = _____ degrees Fahrenheit

E   76 degrees Fahrenheit = _____ degrees Celsius

Q23   Convert the following:

A   400 kcal   = _____ kJ

B   2000 J   = _____ kcal

C   97 mmHg = _____ Pa

D   907 Pa   = _____ mmHg

E   106 mmHg = _____ kPa

F   4.7 kPa   = _____ mmHg

Q24   A patient enters the pharmacy wanting to know his body mass index (BMI). He is 6 feet 2 inches tall and weighs 13 stone 12 pounds. The formula for BMI is weight/(height)^2 for weight in kilograms and height in metres. Calculate the BMI of this patient.

_____

Q25   A patient is 5 feet 10 inches tall. What is the maximum weight in stones and pounds the patient can be to achieve a BMI less than 25?

_____ stone _____ pounds

Q26   A patient has a pCO_2 of 53 mmHg. The normal range is 4.5–6.0 kPa. Is this value within the normal range?

_____

Q27   Nutracel 800 is an infusion fluid for parenteral feeding. The energy content is listed as 3400 kJ/L. How many kcal/L is this?

_____ kcal/L

NOTES

Q28   The temperature of a patient is 98.6 degrees Fahrenheit. Express this in degrees Celsius.

-------------- degrees Celsius

Q29   Wool fat is stated as having a melting point range of 36 to 42 degrees Celsius. Express this range in Fahrenheit.

-------------- degrees Fahrenheit

NOTES

ANSWERS

A1   **A**   0.223 g, 0.000 223 kg, 223 000 micrograms

B   0.032 g, 0.000 032 kg, 32 000 micrograms

C   0.045 6 g, 0.000 045 6 kg, 45 600 micrograms

D   0.000 003 52 g, 3.52 micrograms, 3520 nanograms

E   0.59 micrograms, 590 nanograms, 590 000 picograms

F   1200 micrograms, 1 200 000 nanograms, 0.001 2 g

G   0.25 mg, 250 000 nanograms, 0.00025 g

H   6 mg, 6 000 000 nanograms, 0.006 g

I   1300 g, 1 300 000 mg, 1 300 000 000 micrograms

J   600 g, 600 000 mg, 600 000 000 micrograms

K   0.546 g, 546 mg, 546 000 micrograms

L   0.057 kg, 57 000 mg

M   0.008 67 kg, 8670 mg

N   0.000 250 mg, 0.250 micrograms

O   0.000 000 152 mg, 0.000 152 micrograms, 152 picograms

A2   **A**   0.01 L, 10 000 microlitres

B   0.42 L, 420 000 microlitres

C   2130 mL

D   0.95 mL, 950 microlitres

E   23 mL, 0.023 L

A3   **A**   170 cm, 1.7 m, 1 700 000 micrometres

B   0.078 cm, 0.000 78 m, 780 micrometres

C   0.125 cm, 0.001 25 m, 1250 micrometres

D   2.5 mm, 0.0025 m

E   156 mm, 0.156 m

F   0.64 mm, 0.000 64 m

G   120 cm, 1200 m

H   1300 cm, 13 000 mm

I   0.89 cm, 8.9 mm, 8900 micrometres

J   0.009 056 m, 0.9056 cm, 9.056 mm

A4   A   34.59 g

B   1551.85 g

C   57 150 micrograms

D   9579.05 mg

E   210 mL

F   11.048 L

G   33.813 mm

H   2881.1 cm

I   1 247 377.45 mm

J   103.89 m

A5   4.23 g

A6   1100 mL

A7   0.015 mg

A8   1 microlitre

A9   250 000

A10   10 mg

A11   0.028 g estradiol, 0.014 g norethisterone acetate

A12   10.5 cm

A13   75 L

A14   36 mg

A15   0.225 g

A16   A   3.52 pints, 3 pints 10.4 fluid ounces

B   1.34 pints, 1 pint 6.8 fluid ounces

C   15.4 gallons, 15 gallons 3 pints 4 fluid ounces

     D   10.56 fluid ounces

     E   1 pint, 5.4 fluid ounces

A17   **A**   5.68 L

     B   27.28 L

     C   284 mL

     D   6.25 L

     E   12.1 L

A18   **A**   5.73 pounds

     B   308.7 pounds, 22 stone 0.7 pounds

     C   8.82 pounds, 8 pounds 13.1 ounces

     D   27.12 ounces

     E   2.71 ounces

A19   **A**   17 605.35 g

     B   205.03 kg

     C   53.52 kg

     D   1.08 kg

     E   81 390 g, 81.39 kg

A20   **A**   1.83 m

     B   25.4 cm

     C   13.72 m

     D   33.79 km

     E   1.63 m

A21   **A**   4 feet, 4 feet 0 inches

     B   14.2 inches

     C   382.9 yards, 382 yards, 2 feet 8.4 inches

     D   5.71 feet, 5 feet 8.5 inches

     E   70.7 inches

A22   **A**   60.8 degrees Fahrenheit

      B   213.8 degrees Fahrenheit

      C   99.5 degrees Fahrenheit

      D   –22 degrees Fahrenheit

      E   24.4 degrees Celsius

A23   **A**   1674.7 kJ

      B   0.48 kcal

      C   12 930 Pa

      D   6.8 mmHg

      E   14.13 kPa

      F   35.25 mmHg

A24   25

A25   12 stone 6 pounds

A26   No (7.1 kPa)

A27   812 kcal/L

A28   37 degrees Celsius

A29   96.8 to 107.6 degrees Fahrenheit

3

Calculations involving concentrations

LEARNING OBJECTIVES

Questions in this chapter cover the following:

- expressions of strength (amounts, percentage, ratio and ppm) and converting between the different expressions
- finding the amount of ingredients required to make products of stated strengths
- calculating the amount of product of a stated strength that can be made from a given amount of ingredient

Strengths

Q1   For each of the following decide if the strength is w/w, w/v or v/v:

   A   a 3% solution of sodium chloride in water   ----------------

   B   a 1 in 4 cream containing Betnovate cream mixed with aqueous cream   ----------------

   C   a 10% solution of sugar dissolved in water   ----------------

   D   a 5% solution of alcohol in chloroform water   ----------------

   E   1 g of potassium permanganate dissolved in 100 g of water   ----------------

Q2   Express the following as percentages of 100 g:

   A   12 g   ---------------- %

   B   250 mg   ---------------- %

   C   7000 micrograms   ---------------- %

   D   35 g   ---------------- %

   E   0.0085 kg   ---------------- %

NOTES

Q3   12 mL of glycerol is made up to 80 mL of solution. What is the strength of the final solution as an amount strength and a percentage strength?

-------------- amount strength

-------------- percentage strength

Q4   1.5 g of sodium chloride is dissolved in sufficient water to make a final volume of 60 mL. What is the percentage strength of the solution?

-------------- percentage strength

Q5   10 mL of glycerol is dissolved in sufficient water to make a solution of 55 mL. What is the final strength expressed as a percentage and an amount strength?

-------------- amount strength

-------------- percentage strength

Q6   A patient dissolves two 500 mg paracetamol tablets in 140 mL of water. What is the percentage strength of the solution?

-------------- percentage strength

Q7   One Permitab solution tablet containing 400 mg of potassium permanganate is dissolved in 4 L of water. What is the final strength of the solution expressed as a ratio and a percentage strength?

-------------- ratio strength

-------------- percentage strength

Q8   Complete the following table:

	Formula	Amount strength	Ratio strength	Percentage strength
A	500 mg in 300 mL	--------------	--------------	--------------
B	4 g in 360 mL	--------------	--------------	--------------
C	600 mg in 250 mL	--------------	--------------	--------------
D	1100 micrograms in 10 mL	--------------	--------------	--------------

NOTES

E	130 mg in 6.9 g	---------------	---------------	---------------
F	400 micrograms in 3.2 mg	---------------	---------------	---------------
G	20 mL in 290 mL	---------------	---------------	---------------
H	3.5 mL in 0.672 L	---------------	---------------	---------------
I	200 mL in 3.8 L	---------------	---------------	---------------
J	6.09 L in 13.45 L	---------------	---------------	---------------

Q9   In 1 L of methylated spirit there is 1.5 mg of methyl violet. What is the concentration of methyl violet expressed as parts per million (ppm)?

--------------- ppm

Q10   Express the following as ppm:

A   7 mg in 300 L = --------------- ppm

B   100 micrograms in 4 L = --------------- ppm

C   690 micrograms in 0.95 L = --------------- ppm

D   670 g in 40 000 L = --------------- ppm

E   3 mg in 1 kg = --------------- ppm

Converting expressions of concentration from one form to another

Q11   Salbutamol oral solution has a strength stated as 2 mg/5 mL. What is its percentage strength?

--------------- percentage strength

Q12   Complete the following table:

	Amount strength	Percentage strength	Ratio strength
A	100 mg/g	---------------	---------------
B	20 mg/g	---------------	---------------

NOTES

C   50 mg/5 mL   -------------   -------------

D   400 mg/5 mL   -------------   -------------

E   75 mg/mL   -------------   -------------

F   220 mg/5 mL   -------------   -------------

G   125 mg/5 mL   -------------   -------------

H   120 mg/5 mL   -------------   -------------

I   250 micrograms/mL   -------------   -------------

J   0.3 g/g   -------------   -------------

Q13   Aciclovir cream has a stated strength of 5% w/w. Express this strength as an amount per gram and as a ratio strength.

-------------- g/g

-------------- ratio strength

Q14   Complete the following table:

	Percentage strength	Amount strength	Ratio strength
A	0.8% w/w	--------------	--------------
B	0.3% w/w	--------------	--------------
C	0.02% v/v	--------------	--------------
D	6% v/v	--------------	--------------
E	69.3% v/v	--------------	--------------
F	2.25% v/v	--------------	--------------
G	5% w/w	--------------	--------------
H	10% w/v	--------------	--------------

NOTES

I	20% v/v	---------------	---------------
J	25% v/w	---------------	---------------

Q15   Marcain with Adrenaline contains adrenaline at a strength stated as 1 in 200 000. Express this strength as a percentage and an amount in each millilitre.

--------------- percentage strength

--------------- amount strength (micrograms/mL)

Q16   Express the following ratio strengths as percentage and amount strengths:

	Ratio strength	Percentage strength	Amount strength
A	1 in 4 w/w	---------------	---------------
B	1 in 15 w/w	---------------	---------------
C	1 in 20 w/w	---------------	---------------
D	1 in 25 w/v	---------------	---------------
E	1 in 50 w/v	---------------	---------------
F	1 in 75 w/v	---------------	---------------
G	1 in 100 w/v	---------------	---------------
H	1 in 200 w/w	---------------	---------------
I	1 in 500 w/w	---------------	---------------
J	1 in 1000 w/w	---------------	---------------

Q17   The fluoride in a water supply is 0.9 ppm. What is this as an amount in each millilitre and as a percentage strength?

--------------- micrograms/mL

--------------- percentage strength

NOTES

Q18   Complete the following table:

	ppm	Amount strength	Percentage strength
A	0.7	---------------	---------------
B	1	---------------	---------------
C	15	---------------	---------------
D	500	---------------	---------------
E	2000	---------------	---------------

Calculating the amount of ingredient required to make up a percentage strength

Q19   Nerisone cream contains 0.1% w/w of difluocortolone valerate. How much difluo-cortolone valerate is contained in a 30-g tube?

--------------- g

-------------- mg

Q20   How many grams of sodium chloride are needed to produce 200 mL of a 0.9% w/v solution?

-------------- g

Q21   Ster-Zac Bath Concentrate contains 2% triclosan and to prevent cross-infection 28.5 mL should be put in a bath. How much triclosan would the bath contain?

-------------- g

-------------- mg

Q22   Aromatic Magnesium Carbonate Mixture contains 5% sodium bicarbonate. How much sodium bicarbonate is there in a 10-mL dose?

--------------- g

-------------- mg

NOTES

Q23   Calculate the amount of active ingredient present in the amount of product of stated percentage strength in the table below.

	Amount	Percentage strength	Amount of active ingredient
A	80 g	20% w/w	---------------
B	100 mL	0.2% w/v	---------------
C	50 g	22% w/w	---------------
D	200 mL	5% v/v	---------------
E	50 mL	0.25% w/v	---------------
F	120 g	0.5% w/w	---------------
G	500 g	25% w/w	---------------
H	125 g	0.1% w/w	---------------
I	120 mL	0.125% w/v	---------------
J	10 mL	0.05% v/v	---------------

Calculating the amount of ingredient required to prepare a ratio strength solution

Q24   How much potassium permanganate would you need to make 1 L of a 1 in 1000 strength solution?

--------------- g

Q25   How much sodium chloride is contained in 300 mL of a 1 in 100 solution?

--------------- g

NOTES

Q26   Calculate the amount of ingredient in the products of stated ratio strength in the table below.

	Amount	Ratio strength	Amount of active ingredient
A	100 g	1 in 5 w/w	---------------
B	120 g	1 in 25 w/w	---------------
C	300 g	1 in 5000 w/w	---------------
D	200 mL	1 in 8000 w/v	---------------
E	400 mL	1 in 10 000 w/v	---------------

Q27   How much coal tar solution 2% w/v would contain 140 mg of coal tar?

--------------- mL

Q28   What volume of a liquid of strength 1.25 mg/mL would give a dose equivalent to a 20-mg capsule?

--------------- mL

Q29   You require 90 mg of cocaine hydrochloride. How many millilitres of a 1:400 solution is equivalent to this amount?

--------------- mL

Q30   You require 300 mg of drug x and you only have a 15% w/v solution of drug x. How many millilitres of the solution do you need?

--------------- mL

NOTES

Q31 Calculate the amount of product that contains the stated amount of active ingredient of stated strength in the table below.

	Amount of product	Strength	Amount of ingredient
A	---------------	12.5% w/v	635 mg
B	---------------	6.5% w/w	500 mg
C	---------------	2.5% v/v	70 mL
D	---------------	1 in 3000 w/v	650 mg
E	---------------	1 in 260 w/v	450 mg

Q32 Flumetasone pivalate is soluble 1 in 89 of alcohol, 1 in 350 of chloroform and 1 in 2800 of ether. Calculate the minimum amount of each vehicle required to dissolve 500 mg flumetasone pivalate.

--------------- alcohol

--------------- chloroform

--------------- ether

Q33 Aluminium chloride is soluble 1 in 4 of alcohol. How much aluminium chloride can be dissolved in 1.6 L of alcohol?

--------------- kg

Q34 What is the solubility of an anhydrous chemical if 100 mL of a saturated solution leaves a residue of 25 g after evaporation?

Q35 A tablet coating solution contains 20% w/v of coating. A batch of 500 000 tablets takes 100 minutes to coat at a spray rate of 250 mL/minute. Assuming the coating efficiency is 100%, what is the weight of coating per tablet?

--------------- mg

NOTES

Q36   A patient is dispensed a 10-mL bottle of chloramphenicol 5% ear drops. How much chloramphenicol is there in the bottle? If there are 20 drops in 1 mL, how much chloramphenicol is there in each drop, expressed as micrograms?

--------------- mg

-------------- micrograms

Q37   You dispense a 13.5-mL bottle of sodium cromoglicate 2% eye drops. How much sodium cromoglicate does the bottle contain?

-------------- mg

NOTES

ANSWERS

A1 **A** w/v

   B w/w

   C w/v

   D v/v

   E w/v

A2 **A** 12%

   B 0.25%

   C 0.007%

   D 35%

   E 8.5%

A3 0.15 mL/mL, 15% v/v

A4 2.5% w/v

A5 0.18 mL/mL, 18% v/v

A6 0.71% w/v

A7 1 in 10 000 w/v, 0.01% w/v

A8

	Amount strength	Ratio strength	Percentage strength
A	1.7 mg/mL	1 in 600 w/v	0.17% w/v
B	0.01 g/mL	1 in 90 w/v	1.1% w/v
C	2.4 mg/mL	1 in 417 w/v	0.24% w/v
D	110 micrograms/mL	1 in 9091 w/v	0.011% w/v
E	18.8 mg/g	1 in 53 w/w	1.9% w/w
F	125 micrograms/mg	1 in 8 w/w	12.5% w/w
G	0.069 mL/mL	1 in 14.5 v/v	6.9% v/v
H	0.0052 mL/mL	1 in 192 v/v	0.52% v/v
I	0.053 mL/mL	1 in 19 v/v	5.3% v/v
J	0.45 L/L	1 in 2.2 v/v	45.3% v/v

A9   1.5 ppm

A10   **A**   0.023 ppm

          B   0.025 ppm

          C   0.73 ppm

          D   16.75 ppm

          E   3 ppm

A11   0.04% w/v

A12

	Percentage strength	Ratio strength
A	10% w/w	1 in 10 w/w
B	2% w/w	1 in 50 w/w
C	1% w/v	1 in 100 w/v
D	8% w/v	1 in 12.5 w/v
E	7.5% w/v	1 in 13.3 w/v
F	4.4% w/v	1 in 22.7 w/v
G	2.5% w/v	1 in 40 w/v
H	2.4% w/v	1 in 41.7 w/v
I	0.025% w/v	1 in 4000 w/v
J	30% w/w	1 in 3.3 w/w

A13   0.05 g/g, 1 in 20 w/w

A14

	Amount strength	Ratio strength
A	0.008 g/g or 8 mg/g	1 in 125 w/w
B	0.003 g/g or 3 mg/g	1 in 333 w/w
C	0.0002 mL/mL	1 in 5000 v/v
D	0.06 mL/mL	1 in 16.7 v/v
E	0.693 mL/mL	1 in 1.4 v/v
F	0.0225 mL/mL	1 in 44 v/v

G	0.05 g/g	1 in 20 w/w
H	0.1 g/mL	1 in 10 w/v
I	0.2 mL/mL	1 in 5 v/v
J	0.25 mL/g	1 in 4 v/w

A15   0.0005% w/v, 5 micrograms/mL

A16

	Percentage strength	Amount strength
A	25% w/w	0.25 g/g or 250 mg/g
B	6.7% w/w	0.067 g/g or 67 mg/g
C	5% w/w	0.05 g/g or 50 mg/g
D	4% w/v	0.04 g/mL or 40 mg/mL
E	2% w/v	0.02 g/mL or 20 mg/mL
F	1.3% w/v	0.013 g/mL or 13 mg/mL
G	1% w/v	0.01 g/mL or 10 mg/mL
H	0.5% w/w	0.005 g/g or 5 mg/g
I	0.2% w/w	0.002 g/g or 2 mg/g
J	0.1% w/w	0.001 g/g or 1 mg/g

A17   0.9 micrograms/mL, 0.000 09% w/v

A18

	Amount strength	Percentage strength
A	0.7 micrograms/mL	0.000 07% w/v
B	1 microgram/mL	0.0001% w/v
C	15 micrograms/mL	0.0015% w/v
D	500 micrograms/mL	0.05% w/v
E	2000 micrograms/mL	0.2% w/v

A19   0.03 g, 30 mg

A20   1.8 g

A21   0.57 g, 570 mg

A22   0.5 g, 500 mg

A23   **A**   16 g

      B   0.2 g

      C   11 g

      D   10 mL

      E   0.125 g

      F   0.6 g

      G   125 g

      H   0.125 g

      I   0.15 g

      J   0.005 mL

A24   1 g

A25   3 g

A26   **A**   20 g

      B   4.8 g

      C   0.06 g = 60 mg

      D   0.025 g = 25 mg

      E   0.04 g = 40 mg

A27   7 mL

A28   16 mL

A29   36 mL

A30   2 mL

A31   **A**   5.08 mL

      B   7.69 g

      C   2800 mL or 2.8 L

      D   1950 mL

      E   117 mL

A32   44.5 mL alcohol, 175 mL chloroform, 1400 mL ether

A33   0.4 kg

A34   1 in 4

A35   10 mg

A36   500 mg, 2500 micrograms

A37   270 mg

4

Calculations involving dilutions

LEARNING OBJECTIVES

Questions in this chapter cover the following:

- dealing with dilutions of products and calculating the strengths of the original or diluted product
- calculating the unknown when given information about the original amount and strength, the degree of dilution and the amount and strength of the diluted product
- dealing with concentrated waters
- mixing different strengths together and calculating either the final strength or the amounts of products to be mixed to make a stated final strength
- trituration of liquids and powders when the amount is too small to be weighed

Finding the strength of a diluted product

Q1   Calamine cream contains 4 g of calamine in 100 g of base. If 250 g of aqueous cream is added to the base, what is the strength of the final product, expressed as a percentage?

--------------- %

Q2   300 mL of Pholcodine Linctus 5 mg/5 mL is diluted to 500 mL. What is the final strength as an amount in 5 mL and as a percentage?

--------------- /5 mL

--------------- %

Q3   500 mL of a 1 in 1000 solution of potassium permanganate is diluted to 1 L. What is the final strength as a ratio and as a percentage?

--------------- %

NOTES

Q4 Complete the following table:

	Starting strength	Initial amount	Diluted to final amount	Final strength (percentage)
A	2 mg/5 mL	200 mL	500 mL	-------------
B	300 mg/g	30 g	100 g	-------------
C	250 micrograms/10 mL	5 mL	40 mL	-------------
D	200 mg/5 mL	50 mL	200 mL	-------------
E	400 mg/g	75 g	300 g	-------------
F	1 in 500	25 g	350 g	-------------
G	1 in 200	200 g	300 g	-------------
H	1 in 60	20 mL	300 mL	-------------
I	1 in 4	100 g	500 g	-------------
J	1 in 10	5 g	60 g	-------------
K	40% w/w	50 g	150 g	-------------
L	0.5% w/v	40 mL	200 mL	-------------
M	6.6% w/v	70 mL	210 mL	-------------
N	25% v/v	150 mL	500 mL	-------------
O	0.78% v/v	200 mL	2 L	-------------
P	10 ppm	1 L	20 L	-------------
Q	0.7 ppm	50 g	1 kg	-------------

NOTES

Finding the amount of product needed to be diluted to give a stated strength

Q5   How many millilitres of a 20% v/v solution must be diluted to produce 600 mL of a 4% v/v solution?

_____ mL

Q6   How many millilitres of a 0.2% w/v antiseptic must be diluted to prepare a 1 L solution of 1 in 5000?

_____ mL

Q7   How many grams of an 8% w/w cream must be diluted to produce 150 g of a 2.5% w/w cream?

_____ g

Q8   How many millilitres of Hibitane 5% Concentrate should be diluted with alcohol 70% to produce 500 mL of a pre-operative skin preparation? (The *BNF* states it should be diluted 1 in 10.)

_____ mL

Q9   How many millilitres of Hibitane 5% Concentrate should be diluted with water to produce 2 L of a general skin disinfectant? (The *BNF* states that for general skin disinfection it should be diluted 1 in 100.)

_____ mL

Q10   You are required to make 2 L of hydrogen peroxide (20 vols) and you have hydrogen peroxide (90 vols). How much hydrogen peroxide (90 vols) will you need and how much water will you have to add? (The *BNF* states that 90 vols is 27% and 20 vols is 6% hydrogen peroxide.)

_____ mL hydrogen peroxide

_____ mL water

NOTES

Q11 Complete the following table:

	Starting strength	Initial amount	Diluted to final amount	Final strength
A	200 mg/mL	---------------	200 mL	10 mg/mL
B	2% w/v	---------------	400 mL	2.5 mg/mL
C	4.5% w/v	---------------	150 mL	1.5 mg/mL
D	7% w/v	---------------	1 L	700 micrograms/5 mL
E	0.1 g/g	---------------	200 g	1 in 25
F	1 in 3	---------------	500 mL	1 in 300
G	1 in 4	---------------	250 mL	1 in 500
H	25% w/v	---------------	500 mL	1 in 400
I	0.2% w/v	---------------	250 mL	1 in 5000
J	0.25% w/v	---------------	4 L	1 in 2000
K	1 in 16 w/v	---------------	500 mL	0.5% w/v
L	85% v/v	---------------	425 mL/mL	0.5mL/mL
M	5 mg/mL	---------------	1 L	0.005% w/v
N	5% w/v	---------------	1 L	1.24% w/v
O	0.3 mg/mL	---------------	15 mL	1 in 10 000
P	10 ppm	---------------	5 L	0.5 ppm

Finding the amount of diluent that must be added to give a stated strength

Q12 To what volume would 250 mL of 5% w/v solution be diluted to produce a 1% w/v solution?

--------------- mL

NOTES

Q13   How many millilitres of water should be added to 300 mL of a 3% solution to produce a 2% solution?

-------------- mL

Q14   You are supplied with 50 g of 2% sulphur ointment. How much yellow soft paraffin must be added to produce 0.5% w/w sulphur ointment?

-------------- g

Q15   You have 50 mL of Hibicet Hospital Concentrate and need to make a pre-operative skin preparation. How much could you make and what amount of diluent (alcohol 70%) would you need to add? (The *BNF* states that it should be diluted 1 in 10.)

-------------- mL total

-------------- mL of alcohol 70%

Q16   Complete the following table:

	Starting strength	Initial amount	Diluted to final amount	Amount of diluent added	Final strength
A	400 mg/mL	10 mL	--------------	--------------	20 mg/mL
B	200 mg/mL	50 mL	--------------	--------------	2.5%
C	9% w/v	5 mL	--------------	--------------	3 mg/mL
D	140 mg/mL	2 mL	--------------	--------------	1.4 mg/5 mL
E	10% w/w	80 g	--------------	--------------	4% w/w

Finding the amount of product of a given strength that can be made from an initial stated strength and amount

Q17   How many millilitres of 5% w/v solution can be made from 300 mL of a 30% w/v solution?

-------------- mL

NOTES

Q18   How many grams of a 2.5% w/w product can be made from 50 g of 20% w/w?

--------------- g

Q19   Complete the following table:

	Starting strength	Initial amount	Diluted to final amount	Final strength
A	1 in 5000	1 mL	---------------	0.002%
B	2% w/v	100 mL	---------------	4 mg/mL
C	0.25% w/v	40 mL	---------------	1 in 5000
D	2 mg/mL	22.5 mL	---------------	100 micrograms/mL
E	0.02%	20 mL	---------------	5 ppm

Calculating the initial strength of a product given the final strength and the degree of dilution

Q20   What is the strength of a solution such that 10 mL diluted to 200 mL produces a 2.5% w/v solution?

--------------- % w/v

Q21   What is the initial strength of a product such that 200 mL diluted to 1000 mL produces a 1 in 5000 solution?

--------------- in 1000 = --------------- % w/v

Q22   Complete the following table:

	Initial strength (%)	Degree of dilution	Final strength
A	---------------	50 mL to 1000 mL	1 in 400 v/v
B	---------------	500 mL to 1500 mL	5% v/v
C	---------------	300 mL to 1 L	1 in 2500 w/v

NOTES

D	- - - - - - - - - - - - - - - -	40 mL to 4 L	1 in 5000 w/v
E	- - - - - - - - - - - - - - - -	1 mL to 10 mL	75 ppm

Calculating the initial amount of ingredient in a stated amount that is then diluted in a stated way to produce a final stated strength

Q23   What amount of potassium permanganate must be made up to 300 mL of solution such that 10 mL diluted to 50 mL produces a 1 in 500 w/v solution?

- - - - - - - - - - - - - - - g

Q24   Complete the following table:

	Amount of active ingredient in initial product	Initial amount of product	Degree of dilution	Final strength
A	- - - - - - - - - - - - - - - -	50 mL	5 mL to 500 mL	1:1000 w/v
B	- - - - - - - - - - - - - - - -	500 mL	50 mL to 1 L	0.3% w/v
C	- - - - - - - - - - - - - - - -	300 mL	15 mL to 1 L	1 in 5000 w/v
D	- - - - - - - - - - - - - - - -	100 g	10 g to 150 g	2% w/w
E	- - - - - - - - - - - - - - - -	100 mL	0.5 mL to 250 mL	2 ppm

Calculating dilutions when the final amount changes

Q25   A pharmacist adds 10 mL of a 25% w/v solution of sodium chloride to 500 mL of infusion liquid. What is the percentage strength of the sodium chloride in the infusion liquid?

- - - - - - - - - - - - - - - %

Q26   A pharmacist adds 10 g of 30% w/v calamine cream to 200 g of aqueous cream. What is the percentage of calamine in the final product?

- - - - - - - - - - - - - - - %

NOTES

Q27   A pharmacist adds 5 g of coal tar to 140 g of 6% coal tar ointment. What is the final strength of coal tar expressed as a percentage weight in weight?

-------------- %

Q28   How much zinc oxide should be added to 500 g of base to produce a 5% w/w zinc oxide ointment?

-------------- g

Q29   How much calamine must be added to 100 g of 1% w/w calamine cream to produce a final strength of 10%?

-------------- g

Q30   How much salicylic acid should be added to 680 g of 10% salicylic acid ointment to prepare 15% salicylic acid ointment?

-------------- g

Q31   How many grams of yellow soft paraffin should be added to 500 g of 15% zinc oxide ointment to make a 5% w/w zinc oxide ointment?

-------------- g

Q32   A cream contains 1.5 g of hydrocortisone in 30 g of cream. How much hydrocortisone must be added to make the final product contain 10% hydrocortisone?

-------------- g

Mixing concentrations

Q33   What is the final concentration of glucose solution obtained by mixing 100 mL of 5% w/v with 200 mL of 4% w/v and 300 mL of 30% w/v?

-------------- %

Q34   What is the final strength of ointment when 30 g of 5% w/w is added to 100 g of 8% w/w and 70 g of 21% w/w?

-------------- %

NOTES

Q35   How much 20% solution must be made up to 500 mL such that the final strength is 0.1%?

--------------- mL

Q36   Four equal amounts of 10%, 15%, 25% and 30% solution are added together. What is the final strength of the product?

--------------- %

Q37   What is the percentage strength of alcohol in a product made by adding 300 mL of 20% alcohol to 1 L of alcohol 50% solution?
(assume no contraction)

--------------- %

Q38   30 g of Benzoic Acid Ointment, Compound (containing 6% salicylic acid) is mixed with 60 g of zinc and salicylic acid paste (containing 2% salicylic acid). What is the percentage strength of salicylic acid in the final product?

--------------- %

Q39   What is the percentage strength of a mixture of 300 mL of 40% v/v alcohol with 150 mL of 60% v/v alcohol and 150 mL of 70% v/v alcohol?
(assume no contraction)

--------------- %

Q40   You have two solutions of different strengths. One is 100 mg/5 mL and the other is 300 mg/5 mL. How much of each should be mixed together to produce 500 mL of 150 mg/5 mL solution?

--------------- 300 mg/5 mL

--------------- 100 mg/5 mL

Q41   What is the percentage v/v of alcohol in a mixture of 300 mL of 40% v/v alcohol with 500 mL of 21% v/v alcohol and water to make the final volume to 1 L?
(assume no contraction)

--------------- % v/v

NOTES

Q42   What proportions of alcohol 90% and 50% should be mixed to make a 60% solution? (assume no contraction)

-------------- parts 90%

-------------- parts 50%

Q43   In what proportion should 90% and 30% alcohol be mixed to make a 70% solution? (assume no contraction)

-------------- parts 90%

-------------- parts 30%

Q44   In what amounts should 30% hydrogen peroxide and 3% hydrogen peroxide be mixed to produce 450 mL of a 6% solution?

-------------- mL 30%

-------------- mL 3%

Q45   In what proportions should 50% and 30% alcohol be mixed to make a 45% solution? (assume no contraction)

-------------- parts 50%

-------------- parts 30%

Q46   You are required to produce a 10% glucose solution and you require 720 mL of this solution. You start with two solutions of 50% and 20%. What quantities of each would you mix together?

-------------- mL 50%

-------------- mL 20%

NOTES

Concentrated water calculations

Q47   What amount of rose water concentrate is required to make the following volumes of rose water (single-strength):

	Volume of rose water (single-strength)	Volume of rose water concentrate required
A	25 mL	--------------
B	50 mL	--------------
C	100 mL	--------------
D	150 mL	--------------
E	200 mL	--------------
F	300 mL	--------------
G	500 mL	--------------
H	1 L	--------------

Q48   What amount of chloroform water concentrate is needed to make the following amounts of chloroform water (double-strength)?

	Volume of chloroform water (double-strength)	Volume of chloroform water concentrate required
A	25 mL	--------------
B	50 mL	--------------
C	100 mL	--------------
D	150 mL	--------------
E	200 mL	--------------
F	300 mL	--------------
G	500 mL	--------------
H	1 L	--------------

NOTES

Trituration calculations

Q49   What is the ratio of a trituration containing 120 mg of hyoscine with 3.48 g of lactose?

Q50   What is the ratio strength of a trituration made by combining 0.5 g of drug with 5.5 g of lactose?

Q51   What is the ratio strength of a trituration containing 120 mg of hyoscine with 2.28 g of lactose?

Q52   How many grams of a 1 in 10 trituration are required to obtain 500 mg of drug?

-------------- g

Q53   How many milligrams of a 1 in 10 trituration of drug is required to obtain enough drug to prepare 100 capsules if each capsule is to contain 5 mg of drug?

-------------- mg

Q54   How many grams of a 1 in 80 trituration would provide you with 45 mg of drug?

-------------- g

Q55   A pharmacist is required to make a 1 in 12 triturate of codeine phosphate using lactose as a diluent. He can accurately weigh 120 mg of codeine phosphate. How much lactose will he have to weigh?

-------------- mg

NOTES

Q56 How many grams of a 1 in 25 trituate are needed to make 30 mL of a solution containing 2 mg/mL?

-------------- g

Q57 A prescription asks for three powders each containing 8 mg of propranolol. You decide to make a 1 in 5 triturate. How many milligrams of triturate will you need to make the three powders?

-------------- mg

Q58 You are required to make four powders each containing 500 micrograms of levothyroxine. The minimum weight for a powder is 120 mg and lactose is the diluent used. Calculate the formula for the product and explain how you would triturate to get the required amount of levothyroxine. (Assume you can weigh 100 mg and above accurately.)

Q59 You are making 10 powders each containing 0.0625 mg of digoxin. The minimum weight for the powder is 120 mg and lactose is the diluent. Calculate the formula for the powder and explain how you would triturate to get the required amount of digoxin. (Assume you can weigh 100 mg and above accurately.)

Miscellaneous

Q60 If a syrup is evaporated to 75% of its volume and it originally contained 45% w/v of sucrose, what is the percentage strength of sucrose in the final product?

-------------- %

NOTES

ANSWERS

A1	1.14%	
A2	3 mg/5 mL, 0.06%	
A3	1 in 2000, 0.05%	
A4	**A**	0.016%
	B	9%
	C	0.000 31%
	D	1%
	E	10%
	F	0.014%
	G	0.33%
	H	0.11%
	I	5%
	J	0.83%
	K	13.33%
	L	0.1%
	M	2.2%
	N	7.5%
	O	0.078%
	P	0.000 05% (0.5 ppm)
	Q	0.000 003 5% (0.035 ppm)
A5	120 mL	
A6	100 mL	
A7	46.875 g	
A8	50 mL	
A9	20 mL	
A10	444 mL hydrogen peroxide, 1556 mL water	

A11   **A**   10 mL

       B   50 mL

       C   5 mL

       D   2 mL

       E   80 g

       F   5 mL

       G   2 mL

       H   5 mL

       I   25 mL

       J   800 mL

       K   40 mL

       L   250 mL

       M   10 mL

       N   248 mL

       O   5 mL

       P   250 mL

A12   1250 mL

A13   150 mL

A14   150 g

A15   500 mL total, 450 mL alcohol 70%

A16

	Diluted to final amount	*Amount of diluent added*
A	200 mL	190 mL
B	400 mL	350 mL
C	150 mL	145 mL
D	1 L	998 mL
E	200 g	120 g

A17   1800 mL

A18   400 g

A19   **A**   10 mL

           B   500 mL

           C   500 mL

           D   450 mL

           E   800 mL

A20   50% w/v

A21   1 in 1000, 0.1% w/v

A22   **A**   5% v/v

           B   15% v/v

           C   0.13% w/v

           D   2% w/v

           E   0.075% w/v

A23   3 g

A24   **A**   5 g

           B   30 g

           C   4 g

           D   30 g

           E   100 mg

A25   0.49% w/v

A26   1.43% w/w

A27   9.24% w/w

A28   26.32 g

A29   10 g

A30   40 g

A31   1000 g

A32   1.667 g

A33   17.17% w/v

A34   12.1% w/w

A35   2.5 mL

A36   20%

A37   43.1%

A38   3.3% w/w

A39   52.5% v/v

A40   125 mL 300 mg/5 mL, 375 mL 100 mg/5 mL

A41   22.5% v/v

A42   1 part 90%, 3 parts 50%

A43   2 parts 90%, 1 part 30%

A44   50 mL 30%, 400 mL 3%

A45   3 parts 50%, 1 part 30%

A46   144 mL 50%, 576 mL 20%

A47   **A**   0.625 mL

       B   1.25 mL

       C   2.5 mL

       D   3.75 mL

       E   5 mL

       F   7.5 mL

       G   12.5 mL

       H   25 mL

A48   **A**   1.25 mL

B   2.5 mL

C   5 mL

D   7.5 mL

E   10 mL

F   15 mL

G   25 mL

H   50 mL

A49   1 in 30

A50   1 in 12

A51   1 in 20

A52   5 g

A53   5000 mg

A54   3.6 g

A55   1320 mg

A56   1.5 g

A57   120 mg

A58   100 mg of drug and add 900 mg lactose (T1) then 100 mg of T1 and 900 mg lactose (T2). 200 mg of T2 contains 2 mg of levothyroxine. Add 280 mg of lactose and weigh 120 mg per powder.

A59   100 mg of drug and add 900 mg lactose (T1) then 100 mg of T1 to 900 mg of lactose (T2) then 100 mg of T2 to 900 mg of lactose (T3). 625 mg of T3 contains 0.625 mg of digoxin. Add 575 mg of lactose and weigh 120 mg per powder.

A60   60% w/v

5

Calculations involving formulations

LEARNING OBJECTIVES

Questions in this chapter cover the following:

- calculating the amount of ingredients required from stated formulae
- calculating the amounts required when the formula states either percentages or parts
- calculating the amounts of ingredients required for making emulsions

Formulae

Q1   The formula for Gentian Mixture, Alkaline BP is:

concentrated compound gentian infusion	100 mL
sodium bicarbonate	50 g
double-strength chloroform water	500 mL
water to	1000 mL

Calculate the following and complete the table below:

A   the formula required to produce 100 mL of Gentian Mixture, Alkaline BP

B   the formula required to make 300 mL of Gentian Mixture, Alkaline BP

C   how much mixture you could make if you had 2.5 g of sodium bicarbonate

D   how much Gentian Mixture, Alkaline BP you could make if you had 25 mL of concentrated compound gentian infusion

E   how much chloroform water concentrate you would add if you did not have double-strength chloroform water and wanted to make 1 L of Gentian Mixture, Alkaline BP.

NOTES

	Concentrated compound gentian infusion (mL)	Sodium bicarbonate (mg)	Double-strength chloroform water (mL)	Water (mL) to
A	-------------	-------------	-------------	100
B	-------------	-------------	-------------	300
C	-------------	2500	-------------	-------------
D	25	-------------	-------------	-------------

E   Amount of chloroform water concentrate in 1000 mL ------------- mL

Q2   The formula for Magnesium Trisilicate Mixture BP is:

magnesium trisilicate	50 g
light magnesium carbonate	50 g
sodium bicarbonate	50 g
concentrated peppermint emulsion	25 mL
double-strength chloroform water	500 mL
water to	1000 mL

Calculate the following and complete the table below:

A   the formula required to make 100 mL

B   the formula required to make 150 mL

C   the formula if you start with 4 g of light magnesium carbonate

D   the formula if you start with 60 g of magnesium trisilicate.

	Magnesium trisilicate (g)	Light magnesium carbonate (g)	Sodium bicarbonate (g)	Concentrated peppermint emulsion (mL)	Double-strength chloroform water (mL)	Water (mL) to
A	----------	----------	----------	----------	----------	100
B	----------	----------	----------	----------	----------	150
C	----------	4	----------	----------	----------	----------
D	60	----------	----------	----------	----------	----------

NOTES

Q3   The formula for Chloral Elixir, Paediatric BP 2000 is:

chloral hydrate   200 mg
water   0.1 mL
blackcurrant syrup   1 mL
syrup to   5 mL

Calculate the following and complete the table below:

A   the formula required for 150 mL

B   the formula required for 240 mL

C   the formula (in metric) required to make 1 pint

D   the formula if you have 1.4 g of chloral hydrate.

	Chloral hydrate (g)	Water (mL)	Blackcurrant syrup (mL)	Syrup (mL) to
A	---------------	---------------	---------------	150
B	---------------	---------------	---------------	240
C	---------------	---------------	---------------	(1 pint) = --------
D	1.4	---------------	---------------	---------------

Q4   The formula for Paediatric Ferrous Sulphate Mixture BP is:

ferrous sulphate   60 mg
ascorbic acid   10 mg
orange syrup   0.5 mL
double-strength chloroform water   2.5 mL
water to   5 mL

Calculate the following and complete the table below:

A   the formula required to produce 500 mL

B   the formula required to produce 150 mL

C   the formula if you start with 1 g of ferrous sulphate

D   the formula if you start with 30 mL of orange syrup

NOTES

E   the amount of concentrated chloroform water you would have to use to make up enough double-strength chloroform water for 300 mL Paediatric Ferrous Sulphate Mixture BP.

	Ferrous sulphate (mg)	Ascorbic acid (mg)	Orange syrup (mL)	Double-strength chloroform water (mL)	Water (mL) to
A	------------	------------	------------	------------	500
B	------------	------------	------------	------------	150
C	1000	------------	------------	------------	------------
D	------------	------------	30	------------	------------

E   The amount of chloroform water concentrate in 300 mL of product is ---------------- mL

Q5   The formula for a lotion is:

clindamycin (as phosphate)   0.6 g
propylene glycol   6 mL
purified water   12 mL
isopropyl alcohol to   60 mL

Calculate the following and complete the table below:

A   the formula required to make 100 mL

B   the formula required to make 150 mL

C   the formula if you start with 4800 mg of clindamycin

D   the formula if you start with 28 mL of water

E   the formula if you start with 900 mg of clindamycin.

NOTES

	Clindamycin (as phosphate) (mg)	Propylene glycol (mL)	Purified water (mL)	Isopropyl alcohol (mL) to
A	---------------	---------------	---------------	100
B	---------------	---------------	---------------	150
C	4800	---------------	---------------	---------------
D	---------------	---------------	28	---------------
E	900	---------------	---------------	---------------

Q6   The formula for Calamine Cream, Aqueous BPC is:

calamine	4 g
zinc oxide	3 g
emulsifying wax	6 g
arachis oil	30 g
purified water, freshly boiled and cooled	57 g

Calculate the following and complete the table below:

A   the formula required to make 150 g

B   the formula required to make 450 g

C   the formula if you have 10 g of calamine

D   the formula if you have 90 g of arachis oil.

	Calamine (g)	Zinc oxide (g)	Emulsifying wax (g)	Arachis oil (g)	Purified water, freshly boiled and cooled (g)	Total amount of cream (g)
A	----------	----------	----------	----------	----------	150
B	----------	----------	----------	----------	----------	450
C	10	----------	----------	----------	----------	----------
D	----------	----------	----------	90	----------	----------

NOTES

Q7   A powder has the following formula:

boric acid   7.5 g
starch   12.5 g
talc   50 g

Calculate the following and complete the table below:

A   the formula required for 490 g of powder

B   the formula if you start with 67.5 g of boric acid

C   the formula (in metric) if you start with 10 ounces of starch.

	Boric acid (g)	Starch (g)	Talc (g)	Amount of powder (g)
A	----------------	----------------	----------------	490
B	67.5	----------------	----------------	----------------
C	----------------	10 ounces (-------------- g)	----------------	----------------

Q8   The following is the formula for 100 capsules:

paracetamol   50 g
buclizine hydrochloride   625 mg
codeine phosphate   800 mg

Calculate the following and complete the table below:

A   the formula for 28 capsules

B   the number of capsules and the formula containing 562.5 mg of buclizine hydrochloride

C   the number of capsules and the formula containing 896 mg of codeine phosphate.

NOTES

	Paracetamol (g)	Buclizine hydrochloride (mg)	Codeine phosphate (mg)	Number of capsules
A	---------------	---------------	---------------	28
B	---------------	562.5	---------------	---------------
C	---------------	---------------	896	---------------

Formulae involving parts

Q9   A doctor requires an ointment made to the following formula:

Betnovate ointment   1 part
yellow soft paraffin   3 parts

Calculate the following and complete the table below:

A   the formula for 100 g

B   the formula for 280 g

C   the formula if you start with 75 g of Betnovate ointment

D   the formula if you start with 325 g of yellow soft paraffin.

	Betnovate ointment (g)	Yellow soft paraffin (g)	Amount of ointment (g)
A	---------------	---------------	100
B	---------------	---------------	280
C	75	---------------	---------------
D	---------------	325	---------------

NOTES

Q10   An ointment is required with the following formula:

boric acid   2 parts by weight
liquid paraffin   1 part by weight
yellow soft paraffin   17 parts by weight

Calculate the formula for the following amounts of ointment and complete the table below:

A   100 g

B   250 g

C   30 g

D   the amount of ointment you could produce if you had 7 g of boric acid.

	Boric acid (g)	Liquid paraffin (g)	Yellow soft paraffin (g)	Amount of ointment (g)
A	---------------	---------------	---------------	100
B	---------------	---------------	---------------	250
C	---------------	---------------	---------------	30
D	7	---------------	---------------	---------------

Q11   A cream has the following formula:

salicylic acid   1 part
precipitated sulphur   9 parts
aqueous cream   40 parts

Calculate the amount of ingredients required to make the following and complete the table below:

A   100 g

B   30 g

C   if you start with 3.6 g of precipitated sulphur

D   if you start with 200 g of aqueous cream.

NOTES

	Salicylic acid (g)	Precipitated sulphur (g)	Aqueous cream (g)	Amount of cream (g)
A	---------------	---------------	---------------	100
B	---------------	---------------	---------------	30
C	---------------	3.6	---------------	---------------
D	---------------	---------------	200	---------------

Q12   The formula for a powder is as follows:

aspirin	4 parts
paracetamol	2 parts
codeine phosphate	1 part
caffeine	3 parts

Calculate the following and complete the table below:

A   the formula required to make 100 g of powder

B   the formula required to make 1.25 kg of powder

C   the formula if you start with 500 g of paracetamol

D   the formula if you start with 150 kg of caffeine.

	Aspirin (kg)	Paracetamol (g)	Codeine phosphate (kg)	Caffeine (kg)	Amount of powder (kg)
A	------------	------------	------------	------------	0.1
B	------------	------------	------------	------------	1.25
C	------------	500	------------	------------	------------
D	------------	------------	------------	150	------------

NOTES

Q13   A castor oil emulsion contains 25% v/v castor oil. The primary emulsion is made to the following formula:

fixed oil   4 parts by volume
water   2 parts by volume
acacia   1 part by weight

Calculate the formula for the primary emulsion for the following volumes of emulsion and complete the table below:

A   1 L

B   200 mL

C   if you start with 30 mL of castor oil.

	Castor oil (mL)	Water (mL)	Acacia (g)	Amount of emulsion (mL)
A	----------------	----------------	----------------	1000
B	----------------	----------------	----------------	200
C	30	----------------	----------------	----------------

Q14   For an emulsion containing 30% v/v of cod liver oil, calculate the formula for the primary emulsion for the following and complete the table below:
(cod liver oil is a fixed oil)

A   if the final amount of emulsion required is 300 mL

B   if the final volume of emulsion is 1 pint (express the formula in metric)

C   if you start with 450 mL of cod liver oil.

	Cod liver oil (mL)	Water (mL)	Acacia (g)	Amount of emulsion (mL)
A	----------------	----------------	----------------	300 mL
B	----------------	----------------	----------------	(1 pint) = _____
C	450	----------------	----------------	----------------

NOTES

Q15   Turpentine oil is a volatile oil and is required to be prepared in an emulsion at a strength of 15% v/v. For a volatile oil the primary emulsion is made to the following formula:

volatile oil   2 parts by volume
water   2 parts by volume
acacia   1 part by weight

Calculate the formula for the primary emulsion for the following and complete the table below:

A   if you need to produce 500 mL of emulsion

B   if you need to produce 150 mL of emulsion

C   if you start with 30 mL of water

D   if you start with 15 fluid ounces of turpentine oil (give the answer in metric).

	Turpentine oil (mL)	Water (mL)	Acacia (g)	Volume of emulsion (mL)
A	----------------	----------------	----------------	500
B	----------------	----------------	----------------	150
C	----------------	30	----------------	----------------
D	(15 fluid ounces) = ----------------	----------------	----------------	----------------

Formulae involving percentages

Q16   Calculate the amount of phenol in the following formula:

phenol   2% v/v
water to   30 mL

-------------- mL

Q17   The formula for the product is:

ammonium chloride   5% w/v
raspberry syrup   35% v/v
syrup to   100 mL

NOTES

A   Calculate the formula for 120 mL.

B   Calculate the formula for 500 mL.

C   If you only had 100 g of ammonium chloride, how much product could you make and what would be the formula?

	Ammonium chloride (g)	Raspberry syrup (mL)	Syrup (mL) to
A	---------------	---------------	120
B	---------------	---------------	500
C	100	---------------	---------------

Q18   Cosopt Ophthalmic Solution has the following formula:

dorzolamide (as hydrochloride)   2%
timolol (as maleate)   0.5%

Calculate the amounts of ingredient in 10 mL.

dorzolamide (as hydrochloride)   --------------- mg

timolol (as maleate)   --------------- mg

Q19   An ointment has the following formula:

sulphur   10% w/w
benzoic acid   1.5% w/w
yellow soft paraffin to   30 g

Calculate the formula for the following and complete the table below:

A   30 g

B   100 g

C   250 g

D   if you have 7.5 g of benzoic acid.

NOTES

	Sulphur (g)	Benzoic acid (g)	Yellow soft paraffin (g)	Amount of ointment (g)
A	---------------	---------------	---------------	30
B	---------------	---------------	---------------	100
C	---------------	---------------	---------------	250
D	---------------	7.5	---------------	---------------

Q20   You are required to prepare an ointment to the following formula:

yellow soft paraffin   20%
Betnovate ointment   30%
emulsifying ointment   50%

Calculate the formula required and complete the table below:

A   to make 100 g

B   to make 30 g

C   if you have a 100-g tube of Betnovate ointment.

	Yellow soft paraffin (g)	Betnovate ointment (g)	Emulsifying ointment (g)	Amount of ointment (g)
A	---------------	---------------	---------------	100
B	---------------	---------------	---------------	30
C	---------------	100	---------------	---------------

Q21   Benzoic Acid Ointment, Compound BPC has the following formula:

benzoic acid   6%
salicylic acid   3%
emulsifying ointment to   100%

Calculate the formula required and complete the table below:

NOTES

A   to make 100 g

B   to make 30 g

C   if you have 18 g of salicylic acid.

	Benzoic acid (g)	Salicylic acid (g)	Emulsifying ointment (g)	Amount of ointment (g)
A	---------------	---------------	---------------	100
B	---------------	---------------	---------------	30
C	---------------	18	---------------	---------------

Miscellaneous

Q22   Tisept solution contains chlorhexidine gluconate and cetrimide. A 25-mL sachet contains 0.015% of chlorhexidine, how many milligrams of cetrimide will it contain if the concentration of cetrimide is ten times greater than the chlorhexidine?

--------------- mg

NOTES

ANSWERS

A1

	Concentrated compound gentian infusion (mL)	Sodium bicarbonate (mg)	Double-strength chloroform water (mL)	Water (mL) to
A	10	5000	50	100
B	30	15 000	150	300
C	5	2500	25	50
D	25	12 500	125	250
E	25 mL			

A2

	Magnesium trisilicate (g)	Light magnesium carbonate (g)	Sodium bicarbonate (g)	Concentrated peppermint emulsion (mL)	Double-strength chloroform water (mL)	Water (mL) to
A	5	5	5	2.5	50	100
B	7.5	7.5	7.5	3.75	75	150
C	4	4	4	2	40	80
D	60	60	60	30	600	1200

A3

	Chloral hydrate (g)	Water (mL)	Blackcurrant syrup (mL)	Syrup (mL) to
A	6	3	30	150
B	9.6	4.8	48	240
C	22.72	11.36	113.6	568
D	1.4	0.7	7	35

A4		Ferrous sulphate (mg)	Ascorbic acid (mg)	Orange syrup (mL)	Double-strength chloroform water (mL)	Water (mL) to
	A	6000	1000	50	250	500
	B	1800	300	15	75	150
	C	1000	167	8.3	41.7	83.3
	D	3600	600	30	150	300
	E	7.5 mL				

A5		Clindamycin (as phosphate) (mg)	Propylene glycol (mL)	Purified water (mL)	Isopropyl alcohol (mL) to
	A	1000	10	20	100
	B	1500	15	30	150
	C	4800	48	96	480
	D	1400	14	28	140
	E	900	9	18	90

A6		Calamine (g)	Zinc oxide (g)	Emulsifying wax (g)	Arachis oil (g)	Purified water, freshly boiled and cooled (g)	Total amount of cream (g)
	A	6	4.5	9	45	85.5	150
	B	18	13.5	27	135	256.5	450
	C	10	7.5	15	75	142.5	250
	D	12	9	18	90	171	300

A7		Boric acid (g)	Starch (g)	Talc (g)	Amount of powder (g)
	A	52.5	87.5	350	490
	B	67.5	112.5	450	630
	C	170.1	10 ounces (283.5 g)	1134	1587.6

A8

	Paracetamol (g)	Buclizine hydrochloride (mg)	Codeine phosphate (mg)	Number of capsules
A	14	175	224	28
B	45	562.5	720	90
C	56	700	896	112

A9

	Betnovate ointment (g)	Yellow soft paraffin (g)	Amount of ointment (g)
A	25	75	100
B	70	210	280
C	75	225	300
D	108.3	325	433.3

A10

	Boric acid (g)	Liquid paraffin (g)	Yellow soft paraffin (g)	Amount of ointment (g)
A	10	5	85	100
B	25	12.5	212.5	250
C	3	1.5	25.5	30
D	7	3.5	59.5	70

A11

	Salicylic acid (g)	Precipitated sulphur (g)	Aqueous cream (g)	Amount of cream (g)
A	2	18	80	100
B	0.6	5.4	24	30
C	0.4	3.6	16	20
D	5	45	200	250

A12

	Aspirin (kg)	Paracetamol (g)	Codeine phosphate (kg)	Caffeine (kg)	Amount of powder (kg)
A	0.04	20	0.01	0.03	0.1
B	0.5	250	0.125	0.375	1.25
C	1	500	0.25	0.75	2.5
D	200	100 000	50	150	500

A13

	Castor oil (mL)	Water (mL)	Acacia (g)	Amount of emulsion (mL)
A	250	125	62.5	1000
B	50	25	12.5	200
C	30	15	7.5	120

A14

	Cod liver oil (mL)	Water (mL)	Acacia (g)	Amount of emulsion (mL)
A	90	45	22.5	300
B	170.4	85.2	42.6	1 pint = 568 mL
C	450	225	112.5	1500

A15

	Turpentine oil (mL)	Water (mL)	Acacia (g)	Volume of emulsion (mL)
A	75	75	37.5	500
B	22.5	22.5	11.25	150
C	30	30	15	200
D	15 fluid ounces = 426 mL	426	213	2840

A16   0.6 mL

A17

	Ammonium chloride (g)	Raspberry syrup (mL)	Syrup (mL) to
A	6	42	120
B	25	175	500
C	100	700	2000

A18   0.2 g = 200 mg dorzolamide, 0.05 g = 50 mg timolol

A19

	Sulphur (g)	Benzoic acid (g)	Yellow soft paraffin (g)	Amount of ointment (g)
A	3	0.45	26.55	30
B	10	1.5	88.5	100
C	25	3.75	221.25	250
D	50	7.5	442.5	500

A20

	Yellow soft paraffin (g)	Betnovate ointment (g)	Emulsifying ointment (g)	Amount of ointment (g)
A	20	30	50	100
B	6	9	15	30
C	67	100	167	333

A21

	Benzoic acid (g)	Salicylic acid (g)	Emulsifying ointment (g)	Amount of ointment (g)
A	6	3	91	100
B	1.8	0.9	27.3	30
C	36	18	546	600

A22   37.5 mg

6

Calculations involving doses

LEARNING OBJECTIVES

Questions in this chapter cover the following:

- number of doses and quantity to be supplied for specified dosage regimens
- deciding for how long a specified quantity/volume of medicine will treat a patient
- calculating doses and daily doses using dosages based on a patient's body weight
- calculating doses and daily doses using dosages based on a patient's body surface area
- given specified medicines, calculating doses and the quantity to be supplied for individual patients

Basic calculations involving doses

Note: The following abbreviations are used in this chapter: od, once daily; bd, twice daily; tds, three times daily; qds, four times daily.

Q1 Calculate the number of doses and total volume to be supplied to the patient for the dosage regimens in the table below.

	Dosage regimen	Number of doses	Total volume (mL)
A	5 mL bd for 5 days	---------------	---------------
B	5 mL bd for 7 days	---------------	---------------
C	10 mL tds for 14 days	---------------	---------------
D	10 mL qds for 28 days	---------------	---------------
E	15 mL od for 10 days	---------------	---------------
F	15 mL qds for 28 days	---------------	---------------
G	25 mL tds for 21 days	---------------	---------------

NOTES

H	2.5 mL bd for 7 days	- - - - - - - - - - - - - - -	- - - - - - - - - - - - - - -
I	2.5 mL tds for 14 days	- - - - - - - - - - - - - - -	- - - - - - - - - - - - - - -

Q2 How many days will it take the patient to consume all the medicine for the volumes supplied and the dosage regimens shown in the table below?

	Volume supplied (mL)	Dosage regimen	Number of days
A	30	2 mL tds	- - - - - - - - - - - - - - -
B	50	5 mL bd	- - - - - - - - - - - - - - -
C	60	2.5 mL tds	- - - - - - - - - - - - - - -
D	100	5 mL tds	- - - - - - - - - - - - - - -
E	100	2.5 mL bd	- - - - - - - - - - - - - - -
F	200	5 mL qds	- - - - - - - - - - - - - - -
G	200	10 mL bd	- - - - - - - - - - - - - - -
H	300	10 mL qds	- - - - - - - - - - - - - - -
I	500	10 mL od	- - - - - - - - - - - - - - -

Q3 How many tablets should be dispensed to fill the following dosage regimens?

	Dosage regimen	Number of tablets
A	One tablet every 8 hours for 2 weeks	- - - - - - - - - - - - - - -
B	Two tablets tds for 2/7	- - - - - - - - - - - - - - -
C	One tablet every 6 hours for 1/12	- - - - - - - - - - - - - - -
D	Two tablets qds for 3/12	- - - - - - - - - - - - - - -
E	One tablet bd for 1/52	- - - - - - - - - - - - - - -
F	Two tablets od for 2/52	- - - - - - - - - - - - - - -

NOTES

Q4   Tablets containing 2 mg of prednisolone are available. How many tablets should be dispensed to fill the following prescriptions?

	Dosage regimen	Number of tablets
A	8 mg for 1 day, then 6 mg for 2 days, then 4 mg for 3 days, then 2 mg for 4 days	- - - - - - - - - - - - - -
B	10 mg for 1 day, then 8 mg for 5 days, then 6 mg for 3 days, then 4 mg for 1 day	- - - - - - - - - - - - - -
C	6 mg for 3 days followed by 4 mg for 4 days, then 2 mg for 4 days	- - - - - - - - - - - - - -
D	12 mg for 2 days, then 10 mg for 2 days, then 8 mg for 3 days	- - - - - - - - - - - - - -
E	6 mg for 3 days, then 4 mg for 5 days, then 2 mg for 7 days	- - - - - - - - - - - - - -

Q5   What volume of suspension would provide the correct dose for the following examples?

	Suspension contains	Dose required	Volume of suspension (mL)
A	250 mg/5 mL	200 mg	- - - - - - - - - - - - - -
B	500 mg/5 mL	150 mg	- - - - - - - - - - - - - -
C	600 mg/5 mL	150 mg	- - - - - - - - - - - - - -
D	600 mg/mL	750 mg	- - - - - - - - - - - - - -
E	120 mg/5 mL	360 mg	- - - - - - - - - - - - - -
F	200 micrograms/mL	0.05 mg	- - - - - - - - - - - - - -
G	10 micrograms/5 mL	0.02 mg	- - - - - - - - - - - - - -
H	0.3 mL/5 mL	0.45 mL	- - - - - - - - - - - - - -

NOTES

Q6   What volume of suspension should be dispensed for 7 days of treatment for the examples in the table below?

	Suspension contains	Dose required	Volume for 7 days of treatment (mL)
A	1 mg/mL	2 mg tds	---------------
B	1 mg/5 mL	2 mg tds	---------------
C	10 mg/5 mL	2.5 mg bd	---------------
D	150 mg/5 mL	300 mg qds	---------------
E	250 mg/5 mL	125 mg od	---------------
F	500 mg/5 mL	250 mg qds	---------------
G	200 micrograms/mL	0.2 mg qds	---------------
H	50 micrograms/mL	0.1 mg bd	---------------
I	0.5 mL/5 mL	1 mL tds	---------------

Q7   How many millilitres of injection solution will deliver the required dose for the examples in the table below?

	Injection contains	Dose required	Volume of injection (mL)
A	1 mg/mL	0.5 mg	---------------
B	2 mg/mL	500 micrograms	---------------
C	10 mg/mL	0.05 g	---------------
D	100 micrograms/mL	0.5 mg	---------------
E	100 000 units/mL	25 000 units	---------------
F	150 mmol/L	25 mmol	---------------
G	30 mmol/L	0.015 mmol	---------------

NOTES

Q8   Calculate the total volume or quantity to be dispensed for the examples in the table below.

	Strength of medicine	Dosage regimen	Total volume (mL) or number of tablets
A	240 mg/5 mL	360 mg qds for 1/52	---------------
B	250 mg/5 mL	200 mg tds for 1/12	---------------
C	500 mg/5 mL	750 mg bd for 2/52	---------------
D	10 mg/mL	20 mg od for 28 days	---------------
E	1 mg/mL	500 micrograms od for 10 days	---------------
F	Tablet 1 mg	3 mg tds for 14 days	---------------
G	Tablet 200 mg	400 mg qds for 28 days	---------------
H	Tablet 100 micrograms	0.1 mg tds for 7 days	---------------
I	Tablet 0.5 g	500 mg qds for 1/12	---------------

Q9   Calculate the dose and daily dose for the examples in the table below.

	Patient	Dosage regimen	Dose (mg)	Daily dose (mg)
A	50-kg male	50 mg/kg daily	---------------	---------------
B	60-kg female	45 mg/kg daily	---------------	---------------
C	70-kg male	2 mg/kg daily in two divided doses per day	---------------	---------------
D	65-kg female	10 micrograms/kg in two divided doses per day	---------------	---------------
E	15-kg child	36 mg/kg daily	---------------	---------------
F	12-kg child	25 mg/kg in two divided doses per day	---------------	---------------

NOTES

G	23-kg child	50 micrograms/kg daily	----------------	----------------
H	18-kg child	2 micrograms/kg in four divided doses per day	----------------	----------------
I	0.4-m² child	15 mg/m² weekly	----------------	----------------
J	1.8-m² male	45 mg/m² daily	----------------	----------------
K	1.25-m² female	60 mg/m² bd	----------------	----------------

Calculations involving drugs, doses and individual patients

Q10   An 8-kg child is prescribed alfacalcidol at the recommended dosage (50 nanograms/kg daily). One-Alpha oral drops contain 100 nanograms of alfacalcidol per drop. Assuming one dose per day how much alfacalcidol (in milligrams) will the child be given in 2 weeks and what volume of One-Alpha is required if 1 mL contains 2 micrograms?

--------------- mg

--------------- mL

Q11   A 10-kg child is prescribed 12 mL of cefprozil suspension (250 mg/5 mL) per day in three equal doses. The prescriber needs to know what each dose represents in milligrams per kilogram and the total amount of cefprozil (in milligrams) given to the child each day.

--------------- mg/kg

--------------- mg

Q12   A patient attaches an adhesive patch containing fentanyl, which is released at 100 micrograms per hour. Because pain control is not achieved, a further adhesive patch, which releases fentanyl at 25 micrograms per hour, is attached at the end of 24 hours. How much fentanyl (in milligrams) does the patient receive in total at the end of 48 hours?

--------------- mg

NOTES

Q13   A controlled-release patch is designed to release 60 micrograms of drug per hour for 72 hours. In addition the patch contains 20% overage. What is the total amount of drug (in milligrams) in the patch?

-------------- mg

Q14   A 3-year-old child weighing 15 kg requires furosemide at a dose of 2 mg/kg daily. The only available preparation is oral solution containing furosemide 10 mg/mL. What volume of the oral solution should be dispensed so that the child has sufficient for 28 days?

-------------- mL

Q15   An elderly patient requires 500 micrograms of bumetanide daily for 1 week, then 1000 micrograms daily for a further week. A liquid preparation of bumetanide is available containing 1 mg/5 mL. How much of the liquid preparation should be provided if the patient takes the recommended dose for 2 weeks?

-------------- mL

Q16   A patient with a panic disorder is prescribed citalopram tablets 10 mg each day for 7 days then two tablets daily for the next 7 days. It is found that the patient cannot swallow tablets and so the required dose needs to be transferred to the liquid formulation containing citalopram 40 mg/mL. Four drops of the liquid contain 8 mg of citalopram and is equivalent to a 10 mg tablet. How many drops of the liquid should the patient take in the 14 days and what volume of liquid should be dispensed?

-------------- drops

-------------- mL

Q17   A patient requires the following liquid preparations for 4 weeks of treatment. What volume of each should be dispensed?

haloperidol liquid 1 mg/mL   2 mg tds
pholcodine liquid 10 mg/5 mL   5 mg qds

-------------- mL haloperidol

-------------- mL pholcodine

NOTES

Q18   Co-phenotrope tablets contain diphenoxylate hydrochloride 2.5 mg and atropine sulphate 25 micrograms. If a patient takes four tablets initially followed by two tablets every 6 hours for the next 4 doses, what is the total quantity (in milligrams) of the two drugs taken by the patient?

--------------- mg diphenoxylate HCl

--------------- mg atropine sulphate

Q19   A 60-kg patient requires an injection of 10 nanograms/kg of calcitriol three times a week. The only suitable injection available contains 2 micrograms per millilitre. What volume of injection should be administered to the patient at each dose? If each dose is increased by 500 nanograms for the following week, what is the total amount of calcitriol (in micrograms) given to the patient in the 2-week period?

--------------- mL

--------------- micrograms

Q20   A male patient requires paclitaxel for treatment of Kaposi's sarcoma at a dose of 100 mg/m². 5-mL vials of paclitaxel concentrate are available containing 6 mg/mL. The estimated surface area of the patient is 1.80 m². What dose of paclitaxel will the patient require and how many 5-mL vials of concentrate will provide this dose?

--------------- mg

--------------- vials

Q21   A 3-year-old child weighing 15 kg requires an intravenous injection of alfentanil at a dose of 30 micrograms/kg. Alfentanil injection is available in 2-mL ampoules containing 1 mg of alfentanil. What volume of injection should be given to the child?

--------------- mL

Q22   A prescriber asks if a dose of 10 drops of Niferex elixir three times a day is suitable for a child weighing 9 kg and how much iron in milligrams is contained in this daily dose. What is your answer?

(The recommended dose for a child is one drop per 450 g of body weight, three times a day. One drop contains 500 micrograms of iron.)

--------------- mg iron

NOTES

Q23   A patient requires 980 mg of iron per week given daily as ferrous gluconate tablets. A 300 mg tablet of ferrous gluconate contains the equivalent of 35 mg iron. How many tablets per day should be prescribed for the patient?

--------------- tablets per day

Q24   A child requires 37.5 mg of iron daily. The only iron syrup available is Plesmet, which contains the equivalent of 25 mg of iron per 5 mL. A 150-mL bottle is dispensed. What volume should be given to the child each day and what volume will be left after 14 days of treatment?

--------------- mL daily

-------------- mL

Q25   A child requires 75 mg of chloroquine once a week. Chloroquine sulphate syrup is available containing 50 mg of chloroquine in 5 mL. The child is going to a malarial area for 4 weeks and is required to take the syrup for 1 week before, during and 4 weeks after travel. What is the dose for the syrup and how much should be prescribed for the child to the nearest 10 mL?

--------------- mL dose

-------------- mL

Q26   A patient is prescribed co-codamol (30/500) tablets, three times a day for a week. The patient also takes Nurofen Plus, two tablets three times a day. How much codeine would the patient consume during the course of treatment and is this amount above the maximum *BNF* dose for codeine?

(Nurofen Plus contains ibuprofen 200 mg and codeine phosphate 12.8 mg. The maximum recommended dose for codeine phosphate is 240 mg per day.)

--------------- mg

NOTES

Q27   A 5-year-old child (body surface area = 0.73 m^2) requires treatment with lopinavir and ritonavir oral solution (suitable dose is 2.9 mL/m^2). Calculate the dose (to one decimal place) and the volume of oral solution required to supply the child for 28 days of treatment. For each individual dose of oral solution, how much ritonavir would the child receive? (The oral solution contains lopinavir 400 mg and ritonavir 100 mg/5 mL.)

--------------- mL

--------------- mL

--------------- mg ritonavir

Q28   A 3-year-old child weighing 15 kg requires treatment with stavudine at a dose of 1 mg/kg twice a day. The oral solution is not available and the pharmacist has to make a mixture using 20 mg capsules. The pharmacist makes the mixture to a concentration of 5 mg/5 mL. What volume of mixture is required for 28 days of treatment and how many capsules are required?

--------------- mL

--------------- capsules

Q29   The child in the above question does not like the mixture and is transferred to 'pharmacist made' capsules. The contents of each of these weighs 100 mg (lactose is the diluent) and contains the required dose of stavudine. If the pharmacist makes a batch of 12 capsules, calculate the number of 20 mg stavudine capsules required for the preparation and the weight of lactose required. (The contents of a 20-mg stavudine capsule weigh 40 mg.)

--------------- capsules

--------------- mg

Q30   A child of 6 months (body surface area 0.4 m^2) is to receive zidovudine at a dose of 120 mg/m^2 every 6 hours as an intravenous infusion for 2 days. In the following 3 days the child is given the equivalent dose of zidovudine by the oral route (120 mg by iv route is equivalent to 180 mg by oral route). Calculate the total amount of zidovudine given to the child.

--------------- mg

NOTES

Q31   Calculate the total amount of sucrose a patient will consume from taking one Topal tablet qds for 10 days. Topal tablets each contain 880 mg sucrose. Assuming 1 g of sucrose = 17 kJ, how many kilojoules will this supply of tablets contain?

-------------- g sucrose

-------------- kJ

Q32   How much activated dimeticone (in milligrams) will a child receive if s/he is given 0.6 mL of colic drops tds for 7 days? Colic drops contain activated dimeticone 20 mg/0.3 mL.

-------------- mg

Q33   A brand of vitamin oral drops contains 6000 international units (IU) of vitamin A in 1 mL. Five drops contain 750 IU of vitamin A. If the dose is five drops daily, how many drops are there in 1 mL and how many days of treatment will be contained in a 3.5-mL vial?

-------------- drops

-------------- days

Q34   One IU of vitamin A is equivalent to 0.344 micrograms of vitamin A (as retinol acetate). A tablet contains 0.172 mg of vitamin A (as retinol acetate). If the dose is one tablet daily, how much vitamin A (in IU) will be contained in 21 days of treatment?

-------------- IU

Q35   A child of 4 years is given the recommended dose of 500 micrograms of fluoride ions daily. The child lives in an area in which the water contains 250 micrograms of fluoride ions per litre and the child consumes 3 L of this water per day. Calculate the weekly consumption of fluoride ions (in milligrams) by the child.

-------------- mg

Q36   A child weighing 15 kg requires treatment with sodium picosulfate at a dose of 250 micrograms/kg at night for 14 days. Calculate the total volume of sodium picosulfate elixir (5 mg/5 mL) to be supplied.

-------------- mL

NOTES

Q37   A patient uses Aknemycin Plus solution (containing tretinoin 0.025% and erythromycin 4%) twice a day for 14 days. On each occasion the patient uses 2.5 mL of the solution. What is the total amount of tretinoin in grams and the total amount of erythromycin in grams that the patient will use during the treatment?

--------------- g tretinoin

--------------- g erythromycin

NOTES

ANSWERS

A1

	Number of doses	Total volume (mL)
A	10	50
B	14	70
C	42	420
D	112	1120
E	10	150
F	112	1680
G	63	1575
H	14	35
I	42	105

A2

A	5
B	5
C	8
D	6.7
E	20
F	10
G	10
H	7.5
I	50

A3

A	42
B	12
C	112
D	672
E	14
F	28

A4	**A**	20
	B	36
	C	21
	D	34
	E	26
A5	**A**	4
	B	1.5
	C	1.25
	D	1.25
	E	15
	F	0.25
	G	10
	H	7.5
A6	**A**	42
	B	210
	C	17.5
	D	280
	E	17.5
	F	70
	G	28
	H	28
	I	210
A7	**A**	0.5
	B	0.25
	C	5
	D	5
	E	0.25
	F	167
	G	0.5

A8

A	210
B	336
C	210
D	56
E	5
F	126
G	224
H	21
I	112

A9

	Dose (mg)	Daily dose (mg)
A	2500	2500
B	2700	2700
C	70	140
D	0.325	0.650
E	540	540
F	150	300
G	1.15	1.15
H	0.009	0.036
I	6	0.86
J	81	81
K	75	150

A10   0.0056 mg, 2.8 mL

A11   20 mg/kg, 600 mg

A12   5.4 mg

A13   5.184 mg

A14   84 mL

A15   52.5 mL

A16   84 drops, 4.2 mL

A17   168 mL haloperidol, 280 mL pholcodine

A18   30 mg diphenoxylate HCl, 0.3 mg atropine sulphate

A19   0.3 mL, 5.1 micrograms

A20   180 mg, six vials

A21   0.9 mL

A22   Dose is okay, 15 mg iron

A23   Four tablets per day

A24   7.5 mL daily, 45 mL

A25   7.5 mL dose, 70 mL

A26   1167.6 mg, no

A27   2.1 mL, 58.8 mL, 42 mg ritonavir

A28   840 mL, 42 capsules

A29   Nine capsules, 840 mg

A30   1248 mg

A31   35.2 g sucrose, 598.4 kJ

A32   840 mg

A33   40 drops, 28 days

A34   10 500 IU

A35   8.75 mg

A36   52.5 mL

A37   0.0175 g tretinoin, 2.8 g erythromycin

7

Calculations involving density, displacement volumes and displacement values

LEARNING OBJECTIVES

Questions in this chapter cover the following:

*   the use of density to convert a weight to a volume and a volume to a weight
*   the use of density in calculating the final quantities in formulations
*   the use of displacement volumes in calculations involving dry sterile powders for injection
*   the use of displacement values in calculations for suppositories and pessaries

Basic calculations involving density

Q1   Calculate the weight per millilitre (as g/mL) for the examples in the table below.

	Weight	Volume	Weight/mL (g/mL)
A	22 g	20 mL	---------------
B	27 g	30 mL	---------------
C	147 g	150 mL	---------------
D	0.515 kg	500 mL	---------------
E	0.225 mg	0.25 mL	---------------
F	4800 g	5 L	---------------
G	50 g	48 mL	---------------

NOTES

Q2   Complete the table below.

	Weight/mL (g/mL)	Volume	Weight
A	0.9	15 mL	---------------
B	1.25	100 mL	---------------
C	0.85	0.5 mL	---------------
D	1.1	240 mL	---------------
E	0.95	7.5 L	---------------
F	0.80	---------------	20 g
G	1.2	---------------	150 g
H	0.9	---------------	100 mg
J	1.1	---------------	2.5 kg
K	0.98	---------------	2.94 mg

Q3   Calculate the amount of semi-solid base to be used in the formulae displayed in the table below.

Formulae	Solid Y	Solid Z (g)	Liquid X (mL)	Liquid V (mL)	Base to	Weight/ mL for liquid X	Weight/ mL for liquid V	Mass of liquid X	Mass of liquid V	Weight of base required
A	5 g	0	0	5	25 g	0	0.95	-----	-----	-----
B	6 g	3	2	2	30 g	1.2	1.0	-----	-----	-----
C	200 mg	0	5	0	50 g	0.85	0	-----	-----	-----
D	120 g	60	150	50	1 kg	0.75	1.25	-----	-----	-----
E	500 mg	0	4	12	100 g	0.8	0.9	-----	-----	-----

NOTES

Basic calculations involving displacement volumes

Q4   Calculate the required volume of diluent to be added to the drug powder in the examples below.

	Displacement volume	Concentration of drug required	Amount of drug available	Volume of diluent to be added (mL)
A	0.5 mL/50 mg	4 mg/mL	50 mg	---------------
B	0.3 mL/500 mg	50 mg/mL	500 mg	---------------
C	0.56 mL/g	250 mg/mL	1 g	---------------
D	0.2 mL/250 mg	125 mg/mL	250 mg	---------------
E	0.02 mL/million units	500 000 units/mL	1 million units	---------------
F	0.03 mL/10 mg	2 mg/mL	10 mg	---------------
G	0.05 mL/100 mg	50 mg/mL	100 mg	---------------

Q5   Calculate the volume of water for injections (WFI) required to produce the required injection volume for the examples in the table below.

	Displacement volume	Required volume of injection (mL)	Amount of drug available	Volume of WFI required (mL)
A	0.24 mL/300 mg	5	300 mg	---------------
B	0.7 mL/g	2.5	1 g	---------------
C	0.8 mL/g	5	1 g	---------------
D	0.9 mL/g	5	2 g	---------------
E	0.04 mL/unit	1	1 unit	---------------
F	2.5 mL/5 g	50	2.5 g	---------------
G	0.19 mL/250 mg	5	250 mg	---------------
H	0.3 mL/100 mg	2.5	100 mg	---------------

NOTES

Q6   Calculate the displacement volumes for the examples in the table below.

	Amount of drug	Volume added (mL)	Final volume (mL)	Displacement volume
A	30 mg	4.64	5	--------------/5 mg
B	500 mg	2.2	2.5	--------------/500 mg
C	600 mg	1.6	2	--------------/600 mg
D	30 units	4.9	5	--------------/30 units
E	250 mg	1.8	2	--------------/250 mg
F	1 g	9.2	10	--------------/500 mg
G	1 g	2.3	3	--------------/500 mg

Basic calculations involving displacement values

Q7   Calculate the weight of suppository base displaced by the drug for the examples in the table below. Assume the displacement values have been calculated for the drug in the appropriate suppository base.

	Displacement value	Weight of drug per suppository (mg)	Number of suppositories	Weight of suppository base displaced by the drug (g)
A	0.5	50	100	---------------
B	1.0	50	50	---------------
C	1.5	200	10	---------------
D	2.0	300	20	---------------
E	2.5	100	12	---------------
F	3.0	50	24	---------------
G	3.5	150	20	---------------

NOTES

Q8   Calculate the weight of suppository base required for the examples in the table below.

	Weight of base displaced by drug per suppository (mg)	Number of suppositories	Nominal size of suppositories (g)	Weight of suppository base (g)
A	250	10	1	---------------
B	600	20	2	---------------
C	550	100	2	---------------
D	240	12	1	---------------
E	120	24	1	---------------
F	660	50	2	---------------

Calculations involving drugs and the use of density, displacement volumes and displacement values

Q9   A cream is made to the formula:

zinc oxide   15 g
liquid paraffin   5 mL
aqueous cream to   50 g

The cream is made assuming that the weight per millilitre of the liquid paraffin is 1 g/mL rather than the correct weight per millilitre, which is 0.91 g/mL. What is the difference in total weight between this cream and one correctly calculated?

--------------- g

Q10   A pharmacist wishes to purchase some glycerol. He is offered 2 L or 2000 g for the same price. The density of glycerol is 1.25 g/mL. Which quantity would give him the most glycerol and why?

NOTES

Q11   An ointment has the formula:

methyl salicylate   10 mL
yellow soft paraffin to   100 g

A patient is prescribed 60 g of this ointment. The dispenser assumes that 1 mL of methyl salicylate is the same as 1 g. What would be the actual weight of the ointment if it were prepared using this incorrect assumption? What weight of yellow soft paraffin should have been used in the preparation if the dispenser had used the density of methyl salicylate (1.18 g/mL)?

--------------- g

--------------- g

Q12   A formula to produce 100 g of ointment reads:

oil A   20 mL
yellow soft paraffin   84 g

What is the density of oil A?

If oil A was replaced by oil B (density 0.95 g/mL), calculate the required amount of yellow soft paraffin to produce 100 g of ointment.

--------------- g/mL

--------------- g

Q13   A pharmacist adds 100 mL of water for injections to 20 g of drug Y and obtains 116 mL of solution. What is the displacement volume of the drug per 500 mg and the concentration of this solution in mg/mL? If the pharmacist remakes the injection and starts with 20 g of drug, what volume of water for injections should be added to give a final concentration of 200 mg/mL?

--------------- mL/500 mg

--------------- mg/mL

--------------- mL

NOTES

Q14   A patient requires 500 mL of a 1% solution of drug X. Drug X is available as a vial containing 500 mg of powder for reconstitution. Drug X has a displacement volume of 0.66 mL/g. How many vials of drug X should be used and what volume of water for injections should be added to the drug powder to give the correct concentration?

--------------- vials

--------------- mL

Q15   A patient requires a 6 mL injection of drug Y containing 500 000 units/mL. The drug is available in a vial containing 3 million units as a powder for reconstitution. A doctor adds 6 mL of water for injections to the vial and obtains 7.4 mL of injection solution. What is the concentration of this injection solution? What is the displacement volume per vial for drug Y and what volume of water for injections should the doctor have used to prepare the injection?

--------------- units/mL

--------------- mL/vial

--------------- mL

Q16   A drug is required at a concentration of 160 mg/mL. Drug powder for reconstitution is available with a displacement volume of 0.55 mL/800 mg. How much drug and how much diluent will be required to prepare 20 mL of the required concentration?

--------------- g

--------------- mL

Q17   Drug Z is available in a vial containing 2.5 mg as a powder suitable for reconstitution. A patient requires a total dose of 7.5 mg of drug Z at a concentration of 500 micrograms/mL. The displacement volume of drug Z is 0.1 mL/2.5 mg. How many vials of the drug and what volume of diluent will be required to produce the injection solution?

--------------- vials

--------------- mL

NOTES

Q18 An antibiotic powder for reconstitution with water to produce an oral mixture requires 108 mL of water to be added to produce 150 mL of mixture. If the displacement volume of the powder is 2 mL/g, what weight of powder will be required to produce 200 mL of oral mixture at the same concentration?

-------------- g

Q19 An operator makes 20 mL of a solution containing 125 mg/mL of drug X. The drug is available as a vial containing 250 mg of drug X. The operator uses a displacement volume of 0.21 mL/250 mg. This is incorrect and should be 0.18 mL/250 mg. How much diluent should the operator have used in the preparation and what volume of diluent was used in the incorrect preparation?

-------------- mL

-------------- mL

Q20 A prescription requires the preparation of 2-g suppositories, each one to contain 20 mg morphine sulphate and 200 mg aspirin in a theobroma oil base. Calculate the final formula for 20 suppositories. The displacement values are: morphine sulphate 1.6 and aspirin 1.1.

morphine sulphate   -------------- g

aspirin   -------------- g

theobroma oil   -------------- g

Q21 Calculate the quantities required to produce 50 pessaries to the following formula:

metronidazole   400 mg

pessary base sufficient to produce a 2-g pessary

Assume the pessary base has the same characteristics as theobroma oil and the displacement value for metronidazole is 1.7.

metronidazole   -------------- g

pessary base   -------------- g

NOTES

Q22 A batch of 25 (nominal weight 1 g) suppositories each containing 200 mg of drug X weighs 27.92 g. What is the displacement value of drug X?

Q23 A batch of 50 suppositories (nominal weight = 1 g) each containing 20 mg camphor and 150 mg zinc oxide is prepared in theobroma oil base. Calculate the quantities required to prepare the batch and the weight of each individual suppository.

Displacement values: camphor = 0.7, zinc oxide = 4.7.

camphor   -------------- g

zinc oxide   -------------- g

theobroma oil   -------------- g

weight of each suppository   -------------- g

Q24 Calculate the formula for 20 2-g glycogelatin pessaries each containing 100 mg of miconazole nitrate. The displacement value of miconazole nitrate is 1.6.

miconazole nitrate   -------------- g

glycogelatin base   -------------- g

NOTES

ANSWERS

A1 **A** 1.1

   B 0.9

   C 0.98

   D 1.03

   E 0.0009

   F 0.96

   G 1.04

A2 **A** 13.5 g

   B 125 g

   C 0.425 g

   D 264 g

   E 7.125 kg

   F 25 mL

   G 125 mL

   H 0.11 mL

   J 2.27 L

   K 0.003 mL

A3

	Mass of liquid X (g)	Mass of liquid Y (g)	Weight of base required (g)
A	0	4.75	15.25
B	2.4	2.0	16.6
C	4.25	0	45.55
D	112.5	62.5	645
E	3.2	10.8	85.5

A4 **A** 12

   B 9.7

   C 3.44

	D	1.8
	E	1.98
	F	4.97
	G	1.95
A5	A	4.76
	B	1.8
	C	4.2
	D	3.2
	E	0.96
	F	48.75
	G	4.81
	H	2.2
A6	A	0.06 mL/5 mg
	B	0.3 mL/500 mg
	C	0.4 mL/600 mg
	D	0.1 mL/30 units
	E	0.2 mL/250 mg
	F	0.4 mL/500 mg
	G	0.35 mL/500 mg
A7	A	10
	B	2.5
	C	1.33
	D	3
	E	0.48
	F	0.4
	G	0.86
A8	A	7.5
	B	28
	C	145

D   9.12

E   21.12

F   67

A9   0.45 g

A10   2 L because it weighs 2500 g

A11   61.08 g, 52.92 g

A12   0.8 g/mL, 81 g of yellow soft paraffin

A13   0.4 mL/500 mg, 172.4 mg/mL, 84 mL

A14   10 vials, 496.7 mL

A15   405 405 units/mL, 1.4 mL/vial, 4.6 mL

A16   3.2 g, 17.8 mL

A17   Three vials, 14.7 mL

A18   28 g

A19   18.2 mL, 17.9 mL

A20   0.4 g morphine sulphate, 4.0 g aspirin, 36.11 g theobroma oil

A21   20 g metronidazole, 100 − 11.76 = 88.24 g pessary base

A22   0.58

A23   1 g camphor, 7.5 g, zinc oxide, 46.98 g theobroma oil, 1.11 g

A24   2 g miconazole nitrate, 46.75 g glycogelatin base

8

Calculations involving molecular weights

Basic calculations involving salts and hydrates

Q1 Calculate the molecular weights, the percentage of sodium and the grams of sodium in 25 g of the following sodium salts:

	Salt	Formula	Molecular weight	Percentage Na	Grams of Na in 25 g
A	sodium chloride	$NaCl$	---------	---------	---------
B	sodium bicarbonate	$NaHCO_3$	---------	---------	---------
C	sodium fluoride	NaF	---------	---------	---------
D	sodium potassium tartrate	$C_4H_{12}KNaO_{10}$	---------	---------	---------
E	trisodium phosphate	Na_3PO_4	---------	---------	---------

NOTES

Q2   Calculate the molecular weight, the percentage of iron and the number of milligrams of Fe in 200 mg of the following anhydrous ferrous salts:

	Salt	Formula	Molecular weight	Percentage Fe	Milligrams of Fe in 200 mg
A	ferrous sulphate	$FeSO_4$	------------	------------	------------
B	ferrous succinate	$C_4H_4FeO_4$	------------	------------	------------
C	ferrous fumarate	$C_4H_2FeO_4$	------------	------------	------------
D	ferrous chloride	$FeCl_2$	------------	------------	------------
E	ferrous gluconate	$C_{12}H_{22}FeO_{14}$	------------	------------	------------

Q3   Calculate the number of milligrams of each of the following ferrous salts that will contain the same amount of Fe ion as 200 mg of ferrous sulphate:

	Salt	Formula	Milligrams containing same amount of Fe ion as 200 mg of ferrous sulphate
A	ferrous succinate	$C_4H_4FeO_4$	---------------
B	ferrous fumarate	$C_4H_2FeO_4$	---------------
C	ferrous chloride	$FeCl_2$	---------------
D	ferrous gluconate	$C_{12}H_{22}FeO_{14}$	---------------

Q4   Calculate the molecular weights of the following hydrates, the percentage of water in each hydrate and the molecular weights of the equivalent anhydrous salts:

	Hydrate	Formula	Molecular weight of the hydrate	Percentage of water in the hydrate	Molecular weight of equivalent anhydrous salt
A	ferrous sulphate	$FeSO_4.7H_2O$	---------	---------	---------
B	ferrous lactate	$C_6H_{10}FeO_6.3H_2O$	---------	---------	---------

NOTES

C	ferrous tartrate	$C_4H_4FeO_6.2\tfrac{1}{2}H_2O$	---------	---------	---------
D	sodium sulphate	$Na_2SO_4.10H_2O$	---------	---------	---------
E	sodium potassium tartrate	$C_4H_4KNaO_6.4H_2O$	---------	---------	---------

Q5   For the examples below calculate the amount of hydrated ferrous salt that will contain the same amount of Fe ion as 400 mg of anhydrous ferrous sulphate.

	Hydrate	Formula	Milligrams containing same amount of Fe ion as 400 mg of anhydrous ferrous sulphate
A	ferrous sulphate	$FeSO_4.7H_2O$	---------------
B	ferrous lactate	$C_6H_{10}FeO_6.3H_2O$	---------------
C	ferrous tartrate	$C_4H_4FeO_6.2\tfrac{1}{2}H_2O$	---------------

Q6   Calculate the number of milligrams of sodium and the number of millimoles in 1 g of the following sodium salts:

	Salt	Formula	Milligrams of sodium	Millimoles of sodium
A	sodium chloride	$NaCl$	---------------	---------------
B	sodium lactate	$C_3H_5NaO_3$	---------------	---------------
C	sodium bicarbonate	$NaHCO_3$	---------------	---------------

Q7   Calculate the number of milligrams of magnesium and the number of millimoles in 2 g of the following magnesium salts:

	Salt	Formula	Milligrams of magnesium	Millimoles in 2 g of salt
A	magnesium chloride	$MgCl_2.6H_2O$	---------------	---------------
B	magnesium acetate	$C_4H_6MgO_4.4H_2O$	---------------	---------------
C	magnesium phosphate	$Mg_3(PO_4)_2.5H_2O$	---------------	---------------
D	magnesium sulphate	$MgSO_4.7H_2O$	---------------	---------------

NOTES

Q8   Calculate the number of millimoles in 50 mL of a 5% solution of the following salts:

    A   sodium chloride   -------------- mmol

    B   potassium chloride   -------------- mmol

    C   magnesium chloride   -------------- mmol

    D   potassium bicarbonate   -------------- mmol

    E   sodium bicarbonate   -------------- mmol

Q9   Calculate the number of millimoles of chloride ions in 20 mL of a 5% solution of the following salts:

    A   potassium chloride   -------------- mmol

    B   sodium chloride   -------------- mmol

    C   magnesium chloride   -------------- mmol

Calculations involving drugs

Q10   Calculate the weight of adrenaline acid tartrate (molecular weight = 333) and the weight of adrenaline hydrochloride (molecular weight = 220) that contain the equivalent of 0.3 mg of adrenaline (molecular weight = 183).

-------------- mg

-------------- mg

Q11   Calculate the weight of naproxen (molecular weight = 230) in 500 mg of naproxen sodium (molecular weight = 252).

-------------- mg

Q12   Calculate the amount of amoxicillin sodium (molecular weight = 387) and the amount of amoxicillin trihydrate (molecular weight = 419) that contain the equivalent of 250 mg of amoxicillin (molecular weight = 365).

-------------- mg

-------------- mg

NOTES

Q13   Calculate the amount of isoprenaline base that is contained in 100 mg of isoprenaline hydrochloride and 200 mg of isoprenaline sulphate.

Molecular weight of isoprenaline $C_{11}H_{17}NO_3$ = 211, molecular weight of isoprenaline hydrochloride $C_{11}H_{17}NO_3.HCl$ = 248, molecular weight of isoprenaline sulphate $(C_{11}H_{17}NO_3)_2.H_2SO_4.2H_2O$ = 566.

-------------- mg

-------------- mg

Q14   A pharmacist has to extemporaneously prepare 28 capsules each containing 50 mg of clindamycin. Clindamycin hydrochloride powder is available. Calculate the amount of clindamycin hydrochloride required to prepare 28 capsules.

Molecular weight of clindamycin = 425, molecular weight of clindamycin hydrochloride = 461.

-------------- g

Q15   Topal tablets each contain 40 mg of sodium bicarbonate. Calculate the number of millimoles of sodium in each tablet.

Molecular weight of sodium = 23, molecular weight of bicarbonate = 61.

-------------- mmol

Q16   Algicon suspension contains 50 mg/5 mL of potassium bicarbonate. If a patient takes 10 mL qds for 10 days, what will be the intake of millimoles of potassium?

Molecular weight of potassium = 39, molecular weight of bicarbonate = 61.

-------------- mmol

Q17   A sample of dried magnesium sulphate contains 60% of $MgSO_4$. How many grams of Mg^{++} are contained in a 5 g sample?

Molecular weight of magnesium = 24, molecular weight of sulphur = 32, molecular weight of oxygen = 16.

-------------- g

NOTES

Q18 You are required to make a batch of 25 powders each containing 4 mg of flupentixol. Flupentixol dihydrochloride powder is available. Calculate how much flupentixol dihydrochloride you would require to make 25 powders (assume you are not making an excess).

Molecular weight of flupentixol = 434, molecular weight of flupentixol dihydrochloride = 507.

-------------- mg

Q19 How many millimoles of lithium are provided by 1 g of lithium carbonate and how many are provided by 2 g of lithium citrate?

Molecular weight of lithium carbonate ($Li_2 CO_3$) = 74, molecular weight of lithium citrate ($C_6H_5 Li_3O_7.4H_2O$) = 282.

-------------- mmol

-------------- mmol

Q20 A pharmacist has to provide a litre of approximately 50 mmol/L of Na^+ for use as an emergency oral rehydration therapy. The only available source of Na^+ is a 1-L infusion bottle of 0.9% sodium chloride. What volume of the infusion fluid should be made up to 1 L with purified water to provide the correct concentration of Na^+?

Molecular weight of sodium = 23, molecular weight of chlorine = 35.5.

-------------- mL

Q21 A pharmacist has to prepare a 10 mmol/L Na^+ solution. What quantity of sodium chloride should be used to prepare 200 mL of this solution?

Molecular weight of sodium = 23, molecular weight of chlorine = 35.5.

-------------- g

Q22 Flupentixol injection contains 100 mg of flupentixol decanoate per millilitre. How much flupentixol is contained in 2 mL of the injection?

Molecular weight of flupentixol = 434, molecular weight of flupentixol decanoate = 589.

-------------- mg

NOTES

Q23   Calculate the amount of haloperidol in 50 mg of haloperidol decanoate.

Molecular weight of haloperidol = 376, molecular weight of haloperidol decanoate = 530.

--------------- mg

Q24   You are required to produce a 4-molar solution of a drug with a molecular weight of 60. Twelve grams of the drug are available. If all the drug is used in the preparation, what is the final volume of the solution?

--------------- mL

Q25   Phenytoin sodium has a molecular weight of 274. How much phenytoin sodium will be required to prepare 40 mL of a 0.2-molar solution?

--------------- g

Q26   A 'specials dispensing service' has to prepare 500 1-mL ampoules of clindamycin injection (120 mg/mL). Clindamycin phosphate is available. Calculate the weight of clindamycin phosphate required to prepare the batch of ampoules, assuming no excess is made.

Molecular weight of clindamycin = 425, molecular weight of clindamycin phosphate = 505.

--------------- g

Q27   Medicoal granules are given to a patient for the emergency treatment of poisoning. The treatment regimen is two sachets immediately followed by one sachet every 20 minutes for the next hour. Calculate the number of millimoles of Na and the amount of charcoal that the patient will receive as a result of the ingestion of Medicoal granules.

Each Medicoal sachet contains 17.9 mmol of sodium and 5 g of charcoal.

--------------- mmol

--------------- g

NOTES

Q28   A cardiac patient is changed from Gastrocote liquid to Gaviscon liquid, both at a dose of 10 mL qds. Calculate the increased intake of sodium (in millimoles) by the patient if the patient takes the Gaviscon for 7 days at the correct dose.

Gastrocote contains 1.8 mmol Na per 5 mL, Gaviscon contains 3 mmol Na per 5 mL.

-------------- mmol Na

Q29   A child of 6 kg is prescribed Gaviscon Infant oral powder at the *BNF* recommended dosage. Calculate the sodium intake (in millimoles) if the child is given three meals a day for 14 days and each meal is followed by two sachets of Gaviscon Infant oral powder. Each sachet contains 0.92 mmol of sodium ion and the dose is two sachets tds.

-------------- mmol

Q30   A patient is changed from calcium and ergocalciferol tablets (1 tds) to Calcichew D_3 tablets (1 od). What is the increase in Ca intake (in millimoles) due to the change to Calcichew D_3 if the patient takes the tablets for 4 weeks at the recommended dose? Calcium and ergocalciferol tablets each contain 2.4 mmol of calcium ions. Calcichew D_3 tablets each contain 12.6 mmol of calcium ions.

-------------- mmol

Q31   What is the equivalent weight of betamethasone contained in 30 g of Lotriderm cream? Lotriderm contains 0.064% of betamethasone dipropionate; 0.64% betamethasone dipropionate is equivalent to 0.5% betamethasone.

-------------- milligrams

Q32   A patient takes one calcium and vitamin D tablet twice a day for 28 days. How many millimoles of calcium ion do they consume each day? Each calcium and vitamin D tablet contains 2.4 mmol of calcium ion.

-------------- mmol

Q33   A patient requires 80.5 mmol of phosphate per day for 7 days. Phosphate-Sandoz tablets are available. How many tablets should the patient take per day and how many millimoles of potassium will they consume during the 7-day course of tablets? Phosphate-Sandoz tablets each contain 16.1 mmol of phosphate and 3.1 mmol of potassium.

-------------- tablets

-------------- mmol

NOTES

ANSWERS

A1

	Molecular weight	Percentage Na	Grams of Na in 25 g
A	58.5	39.3	9.8
B	84	27.4	6.8
C	42	54.8	13.7
D	282	8.2	2.1
E	164	42.1	10.5

A2

	Molecular weight	Percentage Fe	Milligrams in 200 mg
A	152	36.8	73.6
B	172	32.6	64.2
C	170	32.9	65.8
D	127	44.1	88.4
E	446	12.6	25.2

A3

A	226.3
B	224
C	167
D	587

A4

	Molecular weight of the hydrate	Percentage of water in the hydrate	Molecular weight of equivalent anhydrous salt
A	278	45.3	152
B	288	18.8	234
C	249	18.1	204
D	322	55.9	142
E	282	25.5	210

A5   **A**   731

     B   758

     C   655

A6

	Milligrams of sodium	Millimoles of sodium
A	390	17.0
B	205	8.9
C	274	11.9

A7

	Milligrams of magnesium	Millimoles in 2 g of salt
A	239	9.9
B	227	9.3
C	413	17.0
D	197	8.1

A8   **A**   42.7

     B   33.6

     C   12.3

     D   25.0

     E   29.8

A9   **A**   13.4

     B   17.1

     C   4.9

A10   546 mg, 360 mg

A11   456.3 mg

A12   265.1 mg, 287.0 mg

A13   85.1 mg, 149.1 mg

A14   1.519 g

A15   0.476 mmol

A16   40 mmol

A17   0.6 g

A18   116.8 mg

A19   27.0 mmol, 21.3 mmol

A20   325 mL

A21   0.117 g

A22   147.4 mg

A23   35.5 mg

A24   50 mL

A25   2.192 g

A26   71.29 g

A27   89.5 mmol, 25 g

A28   67.2 mmol

A29   77.3 mmol

A30   151.2 mmol

A31   15 mg

A32   134.4 mmol

A33   Five tablets, 108.5 mmol

9

Calculations involving parenteral solutions

LEARNING OBJECTIVES

Questions in this chapter cover the following:

- calculating the rate of delivery of a intravenous solution from the dose required
- calculating the time required for infusion and the volume of infusion solution required
- calculations involving syringe drivers as the method of infusion
- calculations involving specific drugs and their parenteral delivery to a patient

Basic calculations for drugs diluted before intravenous infusion

Instructions for the dilution of drugs and their infusion are given by manufacturers and can be found in the *BNF*. There are three main types of instructions for dilution and infusion.

Volume of diluent stated

Q1 Calculate the number of vials required, the concentration of the infusion fluid and the rate of delivery from the information given in the table below.

	Available product	Total dose required	Number of vials	Volume of infusion	Infusion time	Concentration of infusion fluid (mg/mL)	Rate of delivery (mL/min)
A	500 mg per vial	2 g	---------	40 mL	30 minutes	---------	---------
B	1-g vial	1 g	---------	60 mL	30 minutes	---------	---------
C	75 mg/mL in a 5-mL vial	5 mg/kg for a 60-kg patient	---------	100 mL	1 hour	---------	---------
D	250 mg per vial	500 mg	---------	100 mL	30 minutes	---------	---------

NOTES

E	40 mg/mL in a 2-mL vial	3 mg/kg for an 80-kg patient	---------	50 mL	20 minutes	---------	---------
F	1 mg/mL in a 2-mL vial	4 mg	---------	500 mL	2 hours	---------	---------

Concentration of infusion fluid stated

Q2 Calculate the number of vials required, the volume of infusion and the rate of delivery from the information given in the table below.

	Available product	*Total dose required*	*Required concentration of infusion*	*Time for infusion*	*Number of vials required*	*Volume of infusion (mL)*	*Rate of delivery (mL/min)*
A	5 mg/mL in a 2-mL vial	120 mg	2 mg/5 mL	5 hours	--------	--------	--------
B	1 mg/mL in a 1-mL vial	10 mg	500 micrograms/5 mL	2 hours	--------	--------	--------
C	10 mg/mL in a 1-mL vial	50 mg	2 mg/mL	3 minutes	--------	--------	--------
D	2 mg/mL in a 25-mL vial	100 mg	1 mg in 5 mL	4 hours	--------	--------	--------
E	500 mg in a vial	1 g	5 mg/mL	40 minutes	--------	--------	--------
F	0.1 mg/mL in a 5-mL vial	500 micrograms	10 micrograms/mL	20 minutes	--------	--------	--------
G	96 mg/mL in a 5-mL vial	480 mg	4 mg/mL	60 minutes	--------	--------	--------

NOTES

Rate of delivery of the infusion fluid stated

Q3   Calculate the number of vials required, the volume of the infusion and the time for infusion from the information given in the table below.

	Available product	Total dose required	Rate of delivery	Required concentration of infusion	Number of vials required	Volume of infusion (mL)	Time for infusion (minutes)
A	5 mg/mL in a 20-mL vial	200 mg	2 mg/minute	1 mg/mL	--------	--------	--------
B	1 mg/mL in a 5-mL vial	25 mg	250 micrograms/ minute	500 micrograms/ mL	--------	--------	--------
C	2 mg/mL in a 2-mL vial	8 mg	0.04 mg/minute	20 micrograms/ mL	--------	--------	--------
D	96 mg/mL in a 5-mL vial	1440 mg	24 mg/minute	3 mg/mL	--------	--------	--------
E	50 mg in one vial	100 mg	12.5 mg/hour	0.05 mg/mL	--------	--------	--------
F	100 mg/mL in a 10-mL vial	500 mg	2 mL/minute	2 mg/mL	--------	--------	--------

Basic calculations involving the delivery of intravenous drugs

Q4   Calculate the number of drops per minute from the information in the table below.

	Rate of delivery	Number of drops per mL	Number of drops per minute
A	1.5 mL/minute	20	---------------
B	2 mL/minute	20	---------------
C	4.2 mL/minute	20	---------------
D	0.5 mL/minute	20	---------------
E	10 mL/hour	20	---------------

NOTES

Q5   Calculate the rate in mm/hour that a syringe driver should be set at using the information in the table below.

	Required rate of drug delivery	Concentration of infusion solution	Volume of syringe (mL)	Length of syringe (mm)	Syringe driver setting in mm/hour
A	2.5 mg/hour	4 mg/mL	5	60	--------------
B	250 micrograms/hour	1 mg/mL	5	80	--------------
C	100 micrograms/hour	0.2 mg/mL	10	50	--------------
D	2 mg/hour	5 mg/mL	10	100	--------------
E	30 micrograms/hour	0.1 mg/mL	5	50	--------------
F	2.4 micrograms/hour	10 micrograms/mL	2	50	--------------
G	4 mg/hour	10 mg/mL	5	80	--------------
H	120 micrograms/hour	150 micrograms/mL	10	50	--------------

Calculations involving drugs and parenteral solutions

Q6   You are provided with a 10-mL ampoule containing 1.5 g of drug X. The contents of the ampoule are mixed with 5% glucose solution to provide a 0.3% solution of X. This prepared solution is infused into a patient so that they receive 12 mg of X per minute. Calculate the volume per minute to be infused into the patient.

-------------- mL/minute

Q7   You are provided with a 10-mL ampoule containing 50% magnesium sulphate. Before use the ampoule must be diluted with 1.5 parts of water for injections. A patient requires 4 g of magnesium sulphate to be administered as an infusion over 10 minutes. What volume of the diluted injection will provide 4 g of magnesium sulphate and what should be the rate (in millilitres per minute) of the infusion?

-------------- mL

-------------- mL/minute

NOTES

Q8   Magnesium sulphate 50% injection contains approximately 2 mmol/mL. The injection has to be diluted with 1.5 parts of water for injections before use. A patient requires 8 mmol of magnesium sulphate to be infused over 20 minutes. Two-millilitre ampoules of magnesium sulphate are available. How many ampoules will be required to provide the correct dose of magnesium sulphate, what will be the volume of the diluted injection and how many millilitres per minute should be infused?

_____ ampoules

_____ mL

_____ mL/minute

Q9   A 30-kg child requires an intravenous infusion with ticarcillin at a dose of 80 mg/kg. It is proposed to dissolve the contents of a vial of Timentin containing 3 g of ticarcillin powder for reconstitution in 100 mL of water for injections and infuse over 40 minutes. What rate of infusion (in mL/minute) and volume should be given so that the child receives the correct dose?

_____ mL/minute

_____ mL

Q10   A 16-kg child requires an infusion of co-amoxiclav at a dose of 25 mg/kg. It is proposed to dissolve the contents of a vial containing 600 mg of co-amoxiclav in 60 mL of water for injections and give the infusion over 40 minutes. What volume and at what rate (in mL/minute) should the patient be given the infusion?

_____ mL

_____ mL/minute

Q11   A 3-year-old child of normal weight requires an intravenous injection of pentazocine at a dose of 500 micrograms/kg. A 2-mL ampoule of pentazocine injection containing 30 mg/mL is available. What volume of injection should be given to the child? The 3-year-old weighs 15 kg.

_____ mL

NOTES

Q12   An intravenous infusion of pentastarch is presented as a 6% and as a 10% solution in 0.9% sodium chloride. The recommended dose is 2500 mL of the 6% solution and 1500 mL of the 10% solution. Calculate the amount of pentastarch and sodium chloride given to a patient if both the 6% and the 10% solutions are given at the recommended dose.

6% solution

--------------- g pentastarch

--------------- g sodium chloride

10% solution

--------------- g pentastarch

--------------- g sodium chloride

Q13   A 65-kg man requires an infusion of a blood volume expander at a dose of 20 mL/kg in 24 hours. He is initially given an infusion of 500 mL, then the remainder at a constant rate for the next 20 hours. At what rate in mL/hour should the remainder be given?

If the infusion is given via an administration device, which is set at 15 drops = 1 mL, at what rate in drops per minute should the administration device be set?

--------------- mL/hour

--------------- drops/minute

Q14   A concentrate for intravenous infusion of drug X is available as a 1-mL vial containing 5 mg/mL. A 60-kg patient requires a dose of 40 micrograms/kg. This dose has to be infused over 24 hours at a final concentration of 8 micrograms/mL. What volume of concentrate will provide the correct dose and what is the volume of the infusing solution? What is the rate of infusion per hour in micrograms and millilitres?

Volume of concentrate   --------------- mL

Volume of infusion   --------------- mL

--------------- mL/hour

--------------- micrograms/hour

NOTES

Q15   A 50-kg patient requires an infusion of drug Y at a dose of 0.2 micrograms/kg/minute. The drug is available as a powder for reconstitution in a vial containing 2 mg and should be diluted with sodium chloride 0.9% to a concentration of 50 micrograms/mL. What is the volume of the final infusing solution and how long will it take to infuse (give your answer in hours and minutes)?

--------------- mL

--------------- hours --------------- minutes

Q16   An 80-kg man requires an intravenous solution containing 0.5 micrograms/kg/minute of drug Z. The drug is available in a 1-mL ampoule containing 5 mg/mL. Calculate the dose per minute and the final volume of the infusion solution, assuming it will be delivered at 1 mL/minute.

--------------- micrograms/minute

--------------- mL

Q17   A 7-year-old child, weighing 40 kg, requires an infusion of daclizumab at the *BNF* recommended dose of 1 mg/kg. Daclizumab is available as a concentrate containing 5 mg/mL in a 5-mL vial. The required volume of concentrate should be mixed and made up to 50 mL with sodium chloride 0.9% and infused over 15 minutes. How many millilitres of concentrate should be used? How many milligrams of the drug will be infused after 12 minutes?

--------------- mL

--------------- mg

Q18   A child of 12 (39 kg) requires an infusion with tacrolimus (at a dose of 100 micrograms/kg) as part of their treatment for renal transplantation. The required concentration of the infusion fluid is 50 micrograms/mL to be given over 24 hours. What is the required dose and what volume of the tacrolimus concentrate is required (each 5-mL vial contains 5 mg/mL)? What is the volume of the infusing solution?

--------------- micrograms

--------------- mL

--------------- mL

NOTES

Q19   A ventilated intensive-care patient (50 kg) requires an intravenous infusion of remifentanil at a dose of 100 nanograms/kg/minute. The drug is available as a powder for reconstitution in a vial containing 1 mg and should be diluted with glucose 5% to a concentration of 20 micrograms/mL. What should be the volume of the final infusing solution and how many minutes will it take to infuse?

--------------- mL

-------------- minutes

Q20   A 3-year-old child, weighing 15 kg, requires an intravenous infusion with alfentanil at a dose of 50 micrograms/kg over 10 minutes. The drug is available for dilution before use as a 1-mL vial containing 5 mg. If the vial is dissolved in glucose 5% to produce 100 mL of infusion fluid, what total volume and what volume per minute should be given to the child?

--------------- mL

--------------- mL

Q21   A patient requires 200 mg of itraconazole by intravenous solution once daily. The drug is available in a 25-mL vial containing 10 mg/mL. The 25-mL vial is mixed with 50 mL of infusion diluent. How much of the solution should be infused into the patient?

--------------- mL

Q22   Ketamine is available as a 20-mL vial containing 10 mg/mL. It must be diluted before use with sodium chloride 0.9% to a concentration of 1 mg/mL. To induce anaesthesia a 55-kg patient requires a dose of 0.5 mg/kg. To maintain anaesthesia the patient requires 20 micrograms/kg/minute. Calculate the volume of the infusion fluid containing the drug, the volume that should be injected to induce anaesthesia and the total volume that will be required to maintain anaesthesia for 15 minutes.

--------------- mL

--------------- mL

--------------- mL

NOTES

Q23   A concentrated sterile solution of drug X (250 micrograms/mL) is provided for use in a syringe driver. The syringe driver has a capacity of 10 mL and the syringe length is 50 mm. The patient requires drug X at a rate of 100 micrograms/hour. Calculate the driver setting for the delivery of the drug in mm/hour.

_____ mm/hour

Q24   A syringe driver, which has a syringe volume of 10 mL and is graduated to 100 mm, is set to deliver 2 mm/hour of drug Y. The concentration of drug Y in the syringe driver is 10 mg/mL. What is the dose of drug Y being delivered per hour to the patient?

_____ mg

Q25   Drug Z is to be delivered to a patient via a syringe driver at 50 micrograms per hour. The syringe driver has a volume of 5 mL and a length of 50 mm, and is set to deliver 2.5 mm/hour. What is the concentration of the infusing drug solution in micrograms/mL?

_____ micrograms/mL

NOTES

ANSWERS

A1

	Number of vials	Concentration of infusion fluid (mg/mL)	Rate of delivery (mL/minute)
A	4	50	1.33
B	1	16.7	2
C	1	3	1.7
D	2	5	3.33
E	3	4.8	2.5
F	2	0.008	4.2

A2

	Number of vials required	Volume of infusion (mL)	Rate of delivery (mL/minute)
A	12	300	1
B	10	100	0.83
C	5	25	8.3
D	2	500	2.1
E	2	200	5
F	1	50	2.5
G	1	120	2

A3

	Number of vials required	Volume of infusion	Time for infusion
A	2	200 mL	100 minutes (1 hour 40 minutes)
B	5	50 mL	100 minutes
C	2	400 mL	200 minutes
D	3	480 mL	60 minutes
E	2	2000 mL	480 minutes
F	½ vial or 5 mL	250 mL	125 minutes

A4   **A**   30

     B   40

     C   84

     D   10

     E   3.3

A5   **A**   7.5

     B   4

     C   2.5

     D   4

     E   3

     F   6

     G   6.4

     H   4

A6   4 mL/minute

A7   20 mL, 2 mL/minute

A8   2 × 2-mL ampoules, 10 mL, 0.5 mL/minute

A9   2 mL/minute, 80 mL

A10   40 mL, 1 mL/minute

A11   0.25 mL

A12   6% solution: 150 g pentastarch, 22.5 g sodium chloride

     10% solution: 150 g pentastarch, 13.5 g sodium chloride

A13   40 mL/hour, 10 drops per minute

A14   Volume of concentrate = 0.48 mL, volume of infusion = 300 mL, 12.5 mL per hour, 100 micrograms/hour

A15   40 mL, 3 hours 20 minutes

A16   40 micrograms/minute, 125 mL

A17   8 mL, 32 mg

A18   3900 micrograms, 0.78 mL, 78 mL

A19   50 mL, 200 minutes

A20   15 mL, 1.5 mL

A21   60 mL

A22   200 mL, 27.5 mL, 16.5 mL

A23   2 mm/hour

A24   2 mg

A25   200 micrograms/mL